Samoa On My Mind

Also by James Y Hung:

Finding Fat Lady's Shoe: A Memoir of Growing up in Hong Kong and Malaysia (2013)

FOB in Paradise: A Memoir (2014)

Silk Road on My Mind (2015)

Practical Ophthalmology: A Concise Manual for the Non-Ophthalmologist (2016)

The Chinese Language Demystified (2018)

Introduction to Tang Poetry (2019)

Sightless: A Novel (2019)

I Left My Heart in Malaya (2020)

Class of 1964 (2021)

Cambodia On My Mind (2021)

Available through Amazon in paperback and Kindle e-book. E-book also available through Barnes & Noble.

Finding Fat Lady's Shoe

An intensely reflective tale of a family uprooted by war, cast adrift onto a sea of uncertainty.—Kirkus Review

Dr. James Hung's life story echoes others that will probably never be written, and offers a fascinating perspective on Hong Kong's recent past that deserves to be widely read. [4 stars out of 5]—South China Morning Post

FOB in Paradise

Hung has written an absorbing and witty book. Dramatic, nuanced vignettes and vivid descriptions of people and places create a rich tapestry that shows the medical profession at its best and worst.
—Kirkus Review

Silk Road on My Mind

Hung is an endearing mix of benevolence, wryness, and curiosity....there is an appealing Marco Polo-ishness to his project: a boundless wonder for a society unlike his own, not for its differences but for the infinitely recognizable humanity at its center.—Kirkus Review

Practical Ophthalmology

More specialists should create guides of this caliber for nonspecialists. An indispensable ophthalmological volume for any general practitioner's office.—Kirkus Review (featured article 11/15)

The Chinese Language Demystified

An engrossing introduction to the riches of Chinese that should delight casual language mavens and more experienced speakers alike.—Kirkus Review (featured article 6/15)

Introduction to Tang Poetry

...will be accessible to novices and a rich resource for experts.... A compelling, detail-rich resource about Tang verse.—Kirkus Review (featured article 3/1)

Sightless: A Novel

An engaging tale about a singular friendship that gives voice to the struggles of the sightless.—Kirkus Review (featured article 2/15)

I Left My Heart in Malaya

With great tenderness, he recounts the beautiful simplicity of that stretch of his youth...—Kirkus Review

Class of 1964

Hung's prose is clean and leisurely. The book is valuable for the portrait it paints of Hong Kong in the 1960s—a melting pot of cultures, settling refugees, and immigrants from across the world that's fending off the looming menace of mainland China.
—Kirkus Review

Cambodia On My Mind

A sensitive, wide-ranging introduction to a diverse Southeast Asian nation grappling with its past.
... his detailed vignettes, recalling his experiences and inquisitive conversations with everyone from doctors to "tuk tuk" drivers, paint a vibrant portrait of daily life, customs, foods, and challenges experienced throughout Cambodian society.

Samoa
On
My Mind

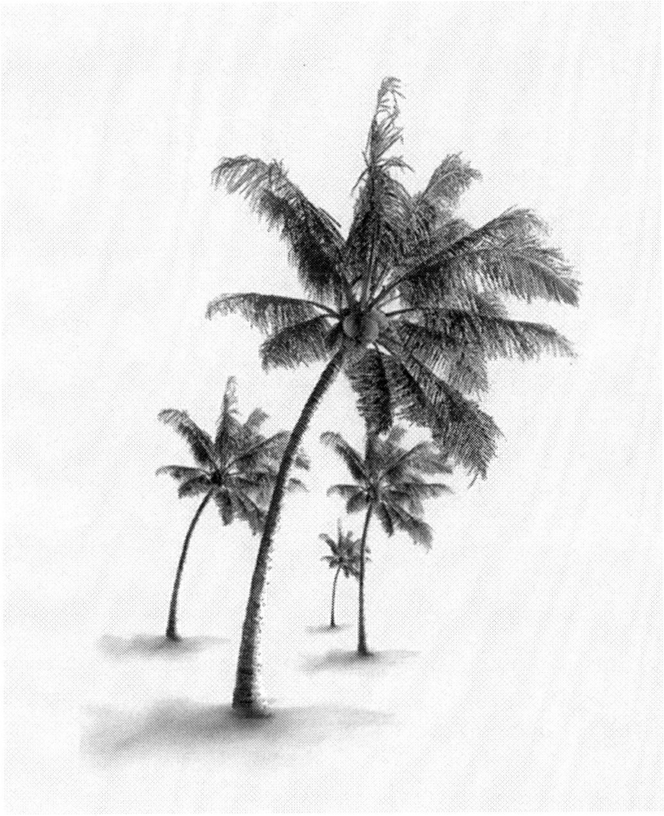

James Y Hung MD

Samoa On My Mind

ISBN: 978-1-7353552-3-8 (James Y Hung)

Edited by Anne Correia

Contents

Author's Note

THIS BOOK IS DEDICATED to my good friend John Fasifilifili Paopao. I got to know the Samoan islands and the people well because of John. If I hadn't gone on those trips with him, I wouldn't have gained the knowledge I did about Samoa and probably wouldn't remember what I did with my life during those weeks—probably just more days in the office. Having been there, I will always remember the good times we had, as well as the good that we did. No doubt we made a difference in the lives of the people we performed surgery on.

Sadly, in early 2020, John passed way from an aggressive form of cancer. He succumbed to the disease a few months after the diagnosis. His family was by his side when he passed away peacefully.

Our friendship lasted over fifty years. Good friends are rare and he was one of those rare good friends. I've enjoyed writing this book, recounting the things we did together. He will be missed tremendously by his family and friends as well as the people of American Samoa and (Western) Samoa.

This is not a travel book. But for those who plan to visit Samoa and/or American Samoa, this book will provide a deeper understanding of the Samoan people and their history and culture.

Thank you.
James Y. Hung MD, FACS, FICS
Honolulu, Hawaii
June 2022

Chapter 1
My Samoan Suite Mate

IN THE SUMMER OF 1970, I returned to Honolulu after a fiasco year at the University of British Columbia in Vancouver, Canada. I had failed half the subjects in my first year of dental school. I don't think I was ever serious about wanting to be a dentist, and the decision to go to dental school was made without much thought.

My four years of college prior to that had been full of excitement and adventure. I spent more time working and playing than studying. Even though I completed the premed requirements, including six chemistry courses, two courses in physics, four biology courses and two courses in calculus, I hadn't majored in science like the other premed students. When I arrived at UBC, I was surprised to discover that I was one of the least prepared in my class.

The 60 medical and 40 dental students took the same basic science courses together. As each course was graded on a bell curve, with the bottom 10% failing, I often found myself in the bottom 10%. I was surrounded by some really brilliant students, especially in the medical school.

But by then I was tired of dental school and was convinced that I wouldn't be a good or happy dentist.

Miraculously, and to my great relief, I was accepted by the University of Hawaii School of Medicine. I packed my bags and left Vancouver and dental school without looking back.

On my return to Honolulu, I purchased a new bright metallic blue Yamaha 90 motorcycle for $350 as my mode of transportation, and rode over to the plush Kahala Hilton Hotel where I'd worked during most of my college years. The personnel director, Miss Jane, who'd hired me almost five years earlier, was happy to see me and said I could start work again the following day.

At the end of the summer, I moved into the residence hall for single medical students in a building adjacent to the Leahi Hospital, which at the time was the main part of the medical school. The room next to mine was occupied by a Samoan. He and I shared a common bathroom.

John Fasifilifili Paopao had gone to Dana College in Nebraska on a full scholarship, returning to Pago Pago afterward to teach high school science. He soon became disillusioned with teaching, and being an excellent painter and sculptor, he thought he would rather work with his hands doing something like surgeries. He made the decision to quit teaching and was accepted to the University of Hawaii School of Medicine not long after.

As we were both outsiders in Hawaii, we quickly became good friends. Neither of us was the gregarious type, and we sort of stayed below the radar in class, keeping our noses to the grindstone.

The head of the pathology department, Dr. Hardman, took a liking to John. He viewed himself as a champion of the Polynesian people. John was only the second or third Samoan ever admitted to a U.S. medical school at the time, and Dr. Hardman was very proud him.

The only other Samoan I knew was a fellow dishwasher when I first arrived in Hawaii. He was over 6 feet 6 inches tall and weighed well over 250 lbs. In contrast, John was my height at about 5 feet 7 inches, and weighed around 160 lbs. He had a lighter complexion compared to most Samoans I'd seen. I later learned that John's father was German or part German. As Samoa was under German rule for many years, there were quite a few Samoans whose ancestors included Germans.

John didn't talk much about his family. I thought he was joking when he told me that he could've been a chief back home, but he declined because he couldn't stand the pain of the extensive tattooing required of a chief. Years later, when I met his family in Samoa, I realized that he was serious.

There wasn't a lot of socializing in medical school. We were all studying very hard to survive. A normal day would be six or more hours of lectures, followed by the same amount of studying afterward. I didn't go out much, but John did allow himself to go drinking every other weekend with his Samoan friends.

One early Sunday morning, sometime around 2 am, I heard a loud noise outside my window. I was half asleep and didn't bother to find out what it was. When I got up for breakfast, I saw that John's window had been broken. I asked him what happened when I saw him later that afternoon, and he said that after returning from a night out with friends, he couldn't find his room key. He said he vividly recalled reminding himself to put the key in a safe place, but he had no idea what he'd done with it. While he was breaking a pane of glass to get into his room, the key was in the briefcase he was carrying! We roared with laughter.

I learned that John loved jokes, and we exchanged them whenever we had a new one. Sometimes he liked my jokes so much that he asked me to repeat them, which flattered me because I knew I wasn't a talented joke-teller, and I often messed up the punchline.

He especially liked my joke about the mechanic: *The mechanic told the owner of a Jaguar that he couldn't fix the squeaky brakes, so he made the horn louder.* Every time he asked me to repeat this joke, we both laughed as if we'd just heard it for the first time. Sometimes we laughed so hard we could barely stand up.

We both survived the first two crucial years—it was generally known that if a medical student got through the first two years, he or she would most likely graduate. For our class, the medical school at the University of Hawaii was only five years old, and it wasn't quite set up for third- and fourth-year clinical rotations yet. Ours would be the last class that had to transfer to another medical school on the continental US to finish med school.

Of the 40 students in our class, I and another student were accepted by the University of Nebraska. John and four others were accepted to Creighton University.

Both medical schools were in Omaha, Nebraska. We even had rotations at some of the same hospitals such as Douglas County Hospital, the VA Hospital and some of the private hospitals.

The winters were cold, but thankfully most of the days were sunny. When I was in Vancouver, many of the days in winter were wet and gloomy, which sometimes depressed me. But in Nebraska, the winter days were generally sunny, and the cold weather in Omaha didn't seem to bother me.

Every month or so, I would invite all the fellows from Hawaii and their spouses or girlfriends to have dinner at our house. By then, I was married.

In the early 1970s, Omaha didn't have any decent Asian restaurants or stores that sold Asian food. I'd been a cook at the University of Hawaii cafeteria for a couple years, so I could cook up some dishes. I usually made noodles and some stir-fry dishes that reminded the rest of the group of Hawaii, using local ingredients and substituting things like angel hair pasta for noodles.

One evening, in the depth of winter, John and I decided to have Chinese food in downtown Omaha. It was snowing heavily, so heavy that we could barely see where we were going, but eventually we found our way to Nam Fong Chinese Restaurant. The Chinese waiter from Hong Kong was happy to see another Chinese person. As I opened the menu, I asked him what he recommended.

He looked puzzled and then a bit embarrassed as he replied, "To be honest with you, I wouldn't eat here. The food here is for white people. By the way, the cook is a black man."

At least he was honest, I thought to myself. By then, John and I were very hungry and didn't know where else to go. I ordered a plate of fried noodle with chicken and bean sprouts, and a stir fry dish of beef and green beans with rice.

When the waiter brought the food, he smiled at me sheepishly. The noodle was the crispy kind called Chung King noodle from a can, and the bean sprouts too were from a can. The stir fry beef with green beans was acceptable and the steamed rice tasted good. John thought the food was great; and in the end it didn't matter where we were or what we ate. We always had a good time together.

In May 1974, we all graduated from medical school. John returned to Hawaii for his internship while I headed for California. Later, John continued his training in plastic surgery in St. Louis, which I understood was one of the best programs in the U.S. at the time, while I stayed in California for my ophthalmology residency and retina surgery fellowship.

After he completed his training, John set up his plastic surgery practice in Hilo, Hawaii, while I stayed in California and began my own private practice. Over the years, we kept in touch with each other. He had married a wonderful woman, Sharon, a nurse he met in St. Louis.

In the early years of our practices, we were both busy with our work and young families. But we maintained contact through occasional letters and phone calls. Later, I visited him and Sharon in Hilo on numerous occasions.

John's background and mine couldn't have been more different. He had grown up on a remote island in the middle of the South Pacific, whereas I had been a city slicker most of my life. As a Chinese, I came from an ethnic group comprised of over a billion people, whereas all the Samoans in the world totaled to less than half a million. In his islands of American Samoa, the entire population was less than 70,000. In Hong Kong, one single housing project would have as many people.

I sometimes imagined that he must feel very special, belonging to truly a minority group. In my case, there were so many of us that even if I were one in a million in the Chinese race, there would still be over a thousand of us!

In spite of our differences John and I got along very well, and we maintained an easy friendship over the years.

Chapter 2

To American Samoa: John's Account

IN 2004, I WENT ON MY FIRST TRIP TO AMERICAN SAMOA. John and a few physicians from Hilo and Honolulu had made the trip before, but at the time I was busy with my own projects in Guilin in Southeast China, Urumqi in Northwest China, and Cambodia, and I hadn't been able to make the trip then. This chapter is John's verbatim account of our 2004 trip.

The group consisted of John and his wife, Sharon, me, and Doug Johnson, a dermatologist in Honolulu who, like me, also happened to be a graduate of the University of Nebraska Medical School. Doug was a native Nebraskan. Two other doctors also joined our party—Steve Garon, an anesthesiologist from Hilo, and Tom Namiki, a pathologist from Honolulu.

"Kimo" in the narration refers to me. This name, which in Hawaiian means James, was given to me by a Hawaiian professor at the medical school, Dr. Richard K. Blaisdell.

Dr. Richard Kekuni Akana Blaisdell was the founding chairperson of the department of medicine of John A. Burns School of Medicine at the University of Hawaii and a prominent Hawaii sovereignty activist. He was already a sovereignty activist when I met him in the 1970s, though not yet openly. He decided that I should have a Hawaiian name, Kimo, which I'm very fond of and which makes me feel like a true local. Because of my large eyes and wavy black hair, I can sometimes be mistaken as part Hawaiian, which I'm also very proud of.

Dr. Blaisdell took a special liking to John as well and indicated that Samoa should be very proud of John's achievement.

From John's narration of our trip, it's obvious he was a very gifted and humorous storyteller.

Note: the account contains some medical terms and local jargon that may be unfamiliar to some readers, but I've chosen to leave his words as he wrote them, as I feel they add to the story and present an authentic picture of John's character. John refers to himself in the third person.

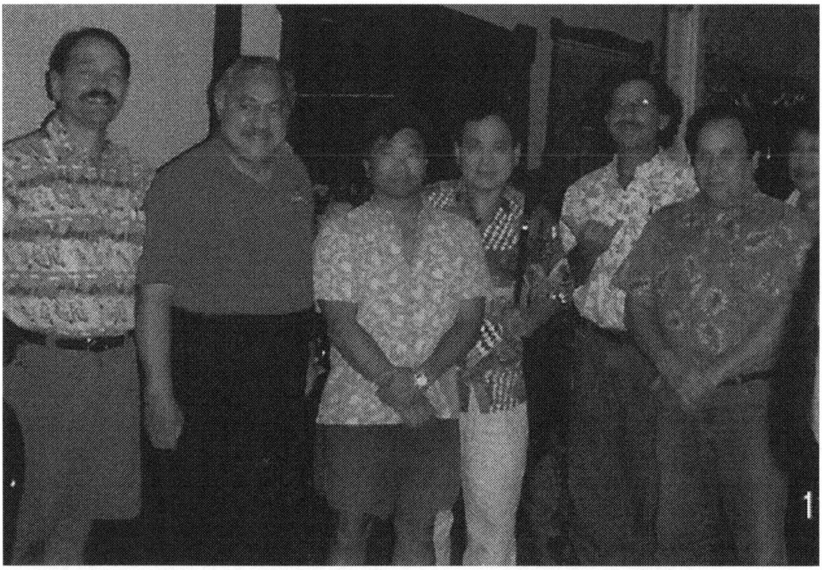

From left to right: Dr. Douglas Johnson (dermatologist), administrator Dr. Joe, Dr. Tom Namiki (pathologist), author, Dr. Steve Garon (anesthesiologist), and Dr. John Paopao (plastic surgeon).

TALOFA MISSION TO AMERICAN SAMOA
11/5/2004 to 11/13/2004

Friday, November 5

Sharon, John, and Steve checked out at Hilo Airport on our way to Honolulu. Steve Garon requests a window on the Honolulu to Pago Pago flight. After he left, John approached the agent and told him to make sure there would be a 300-pound Samoan next to him so that he cannot move in any direction for 5 hours. At Honolulu International Kimo showed up at the departing gate. John was paged and was told to report to the front checkout for Aloha Airlines. After several minutes of mass confusion, John finally met WALDO (Douglas) without his striped shirt. He was standing about 5 yards away. He showed up at the airport without his passport, thinking that he was going to America. While his wife was coming to the airport to deliver his passport, Tom in the meantime was jumping hoops at the airport like O.J. Simpson to get to the boarding gate. This is not unusual as being late to the gate is the usual custom for Tom. Eventually, Aloha Airlines took off to Pago Pago without Douglas. After some *pilikia* at the airport, Douglas finally was able to secure a plane seat with the Hawaiian Airlines flight to Pago Pago some 2-3 hours later. Fortunately, there was no further expense to him thanks to one of his patients who was on duty at the time. On arrival at about 8 o'clock at night Joe, Chairman of the LBJ Board of Directors, showed up at the baggage claim area and hastened our exit, bypassing the customs agents altogether. Outside the terminal we met Sai (John's sister), Vic (assistant medical director) and the Tradewinds Hotel transportation. At this point, John asked Vic that we need some transportation, preferably the same van that they used for transportation of psychiatric patients as we used in the previous year. He was told that we have a total of six psychiatric subjects that need transportation for the next eight days. The rooms at the hotel were quite comfortable.

Saturday, November 6, 2004

This eventful day started out with a buffet breakfast at the hotel's Equator Restaurant. Instead of a van the team got a Toyota 4Runner. Following breakfast, the team headed to town. Sharon was dropped off with Sai, at her work place. The rest of the team went directly to the National Park on the North Shore of the Island in the village of *Vatia.* At the end of the road, we walked for about 50-75 yards with the hope that this will satisfy Douglas' appetite for hiking. This turned out not to be the case as Douglas' ambitions were fueled after we met two other visitors at the Park. In fact, he was given detailed hiking instructions with maps.

From Vatia we headed further East to the village of *Auto*. John dropped off some gifts for family members. For the next three hours we parked at the beach and were delivered a cooler full of oversized *vailima* beers. Chips and ripe bananas later arrived at the scene. Just as we were preparing to leave the area, Tom`s blood pressure dropped below syncopal level. Douglas (a former center with the University of Nebraska Cornhuskers) started the feet raising procedure. John gave Tom a sternal knuckle rub. Tom promptly woke up without further intervention. For a while, Douglas looked like an orthopod with his straight leg raising technique. Steve was very happy that his services were not necessary. Tom immediately declared that he will limit his *vailima* consumption to the pediatric bottle from here forward.

Heading to town, we turned up the hill at Pago Pago Bay to the village of *Fagasa* on the other side of the island.

Coming back, Douglas insisted to be dropped off at the hiking starting area (mafa). He even threatened jumping off the vehicle if his request was not granted. So we reluctantly let him off and he committed this crime by himself under the influence. The rest of the remaining team members returned to the hotel. Three hours later, John, Steve, and Tom returned to the *mafa* to pick up Douglas. Douglas was found sitting on a Tongan-made stonewall sober, pale, wet, with dirty socks from rapidly approaching fog and rain on the National Park mountaintops. He was assisted to the 4Runner and was promptly hydrated with another cold, oversized *vailima* on our way to the hotel. (This is known as drinking on the road.) His color promptly retuned with this oral hydration. Douglas apparently enjoyed his visitation with the birds on the mountaintop. The day was capped with dinner at the Equator Restaurant. Sharon witnessed the normal pulse for the entire team in the upright and sitting position.

Sunday, November 7

Kimo, John, and Sharon went to church at 7:30 a.m. The three other sinners slept late. At about midmorning, the entire team left to pick up To'ona'i (Sunday brunch) at a local store. Next destination, *Nu'uuli Beach.* At the hotel Steve. Tom, and Douglas decided to go play golf. John and Sharon decided to watch football (yes, Rams vs Patriots), and Kimo decided to stay at the hotel and had *ava* alone. After nine holes Douglas made a gruesome discovery. There were no *vailima* beers in the cooler. (John had removed the leftover *vailima* for Sunday football.) Tom was sent away for *vailima.* He discovered that liquor is not sold on Sunday. Nevertheless, he was able to skillfully negotiate an under-the-table transaction with a Korean store owner and proceeded to smuggle adult *vailimas* out of the store.

Monday, November 8

The threat of working finally arrived. The day started out with breakfast at Equator Restaurant. The team went to the hospital. Sharon went with Sai. John and Steve had our clinics at the ENT section at LJB Hospital. Steve evaluated pediatric plastic surgical cases for the next two days. Tom and Douglas had their clinic at the medical outpatient section. Kimo worked with local ophthalmologist Dr. Oo. It was a long day for everybody. Dinner was at Hong Kong Restaurant, hosted by Eni Faleomavaega, American Samoa Representative to the U.S. Congress in Washington, D.C. As a sidebar, he records old traditional Samoan songs. He brought a CD with him which was played "in situ" during dinner. The multiple-course dinner was left up to Kimo for final evaluation and grading. Being a native of Hong Kong, he returned the grade as being relatively acceptable under the circumstances.

Tuesday, November 9

Surgery started for John and Steve. We operated on a 1-year-old James who presented with a long, blond, well-groomed hair with bilateral cleft lip and palate deformity, with an overprojecting, free-floating premaxilla with a very short columella. Fortunately, with Steve's muscle relaxants we were able to close the defect with a relatively reasonable result. Doug and Tom were late. Steve, John, and Kimo split for *Uutulei Beach* with *vailima*-refilled cooler in the trunk. After an hour, we returned to the hospital to pick up Tom and Douglas. That evening, Doug went to dinner with a Samoan friend. Steve, Tom, John, and Sharon went to Kentucky Fried Chicken for dinner. Kimo opted to stay back in his room, have crackers and drink *ava* (without supervision). Under the influence of Kentucky Fried Chicken, Steve and John initiated the investigation into the length of dermatology consultation. We thought that it should be:

1) Scrape the skin.
2) Microscope examination.
3) Prescription for the 2% cream.

This should take a total of about 8½ minutes instead of half an hour. Tom came forth with an explanation to the long consultations. "We talk to patients." This is unreal coming from a pathologist. John and Steve thought that this was <u>outside</u> the normal standard of care. Not supposed to talk to patients. Sharon later reported the rumor about "drunken" doctors with disorderly behavior (like feet raising) at *Auto Beach* three days earlier. These rumors were disseminated by the very people who provided the cooler full of *vailima*. Sharon quickly came to the team's defense, stating that it was an ongoing resuscitation at the time, and that the Hawaii doctors were fully sober, conscious, and upright at dinnertime that day.

Wednesday, November 10

The team left early for LBJ Hospital. Kimo and Douglas did presentations at the conference. Kimo talked about laser treatment of diabetic retinopathy. Doug talked about patients that he and Tom had seen two previous days and were recorded on his digital camera. His presentation was an impressive improvement compared to John and Tom's open-book dermatology practice the summer before on *Savai'i*. John was happy to finally hear the 2% cream towards the end of Doug's presentation. We were all well informed by the two powerful presentations. Our respective clinics and surgery followed that conference. Later that evening, we reluctantly had dinner once again at the hotel's Equator Restaurant.

Thursday, November 11 (Veteran's Day)

This was a holiday in American Samoa, and all the clinics were closed. Doug took off to play golf with a local patient friend at 7:30 a.m. John, Steve, and Kimo went to play golf with Dr. Tui from ENT later that morning. Tom was now experiencing some side effects of previous dinner at the Equator Restaurant and elected to stay back. At the golf course we discovered that there were no carts available. As a result, Steve, John, Tui, and Kimo walked the first 9 holes. The sun was quite hot. Kimo retreated rapidly to the club house after the first two holes and assumed the horizontal position. John and Steve started to develop blurred vision, diplopia and floating spots. (Now without the ophthalmologist.) This rapidly improved with hydration and an upgrade to a golf cart for the second 9 holes. At 6:30 p.m. that evening we went for a buffet dinner at Saddie's Restaurant at the invitation of Big John and Talo. Food was good. A miniature Aggie Gray's Hotel type show then followed at 8:30. At about that time, John and Sharon departed to attend John's high school class reunion. Under the influence of the local *kanaka kava* Sharon's inhibitions were suppressed to the point that she even made a short thank you speech with the microphone.

Friday, November 12

Clinics and surgery resumed. A luncheon for the team occurred around noon. Kimo had a short, violent outburst when he saw somebody remove the pig from the central table. Actually, it was taken out for carving. Joe made a thank you speech to the team, followed by a "wahoo presentation." Clinics resumed thereafter. Steve and John started packing equipment after a couple of procedures. Tom and Doug continued to work late into the afternoon. They were later picked up and the entire team proceeded to *Auto* for a local extended family party. After feasting, spontaneous dancing broke out with Doug being the master of the electric slide. Steve competed with a 70-year-old Samoan man for the "Siva Award" while Kimo rocked on!!

Saturday, November 13

The day started with a buffet breakfast at the Equator Restaurant. Followed by shopping. We then proceeded to town to see the local museum where there is an exhibit of traditional Samoan way of treating skin diseases with local plants. Sharon posed the question, "How does one get *lafa* (ringworm)." Doug's answer, "Sleeping with a Samoan." She then asked the question, "How does one get fungus infection of the fingers." Doug's answer, "Sleeping with a *palaga*." This turned out to be a wash as neither Sharon nor John has either. We then moved on again to *Auto Beach* where we spent the rest of the afternoon. Packing the catch (cases of wahoo) was the next item on the agenda. After checking out we decided to have dinner at the Equator Restaurant once again. This was probably the worst judgment for the entire trip. The quality of the food declined from bad to worse despite a protracted preparation time. John's order of Korean *kalbi* turned out to be a series of circular bones connected by a fibrotendinous-appearing unit, cold as can be. Doug played it safe by ordering a salad that he previously had experience with. Kimo started talking to himself in Chinese about his hamburger.

At the airport, we met up once again with Joe, a representative from the hospital. He started talking about the old Samoan way of treating patients with psychotic episodes. The Samoan's *kahuna* or in this case an exorcist, picks at the demon (*aiku*) who is the one speaking through the patient. So, to exorcise this demon, the people cover the patient with old, dirty rugs and then start the beating on the patient. The LBJ Hospital will have a hard time collecting their Medicare claims if Medicare knows about this treatment, and especially if it is effective. Joe's reply—"The *aikus* are all afraid of light and, therefore, all left *Tutuila* for *Ofu* and *Savai'i* where there is minimal amount of light." We had a great time laughing about this old type of stories from Joe and Big John. Soon thereafter, we saw our plane taxiing to the terminal, following its arrival from Rarotonga. We were given departing leis, said good bye to family and friends, and we were off on our way back to Hawaii. We worked hard and played somewhat hard. The people of American Samoa appreciated our services.

This document will self-destruct in 5 seconds. If it doesn't, you may burn it manually.

Tofa Soifua

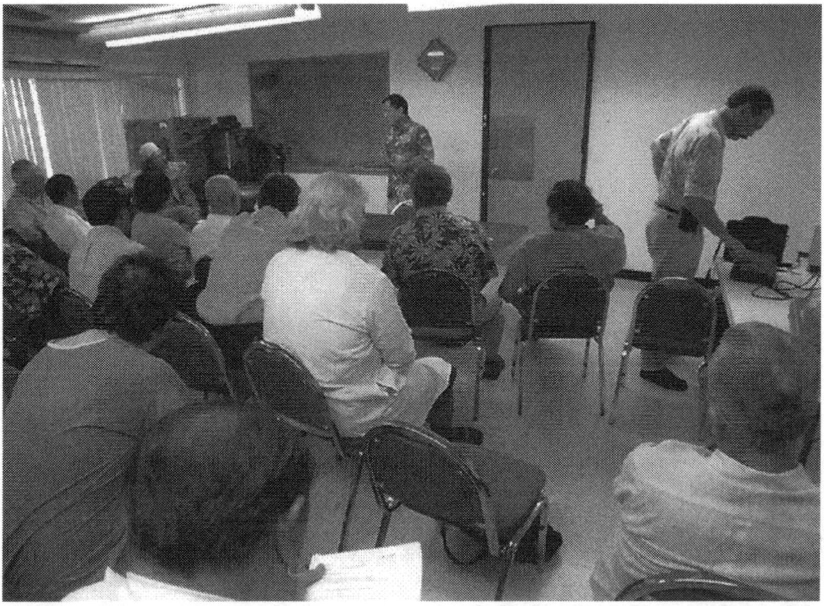

Giving a lecture on the treatment of diabetic retinopathy with laser.

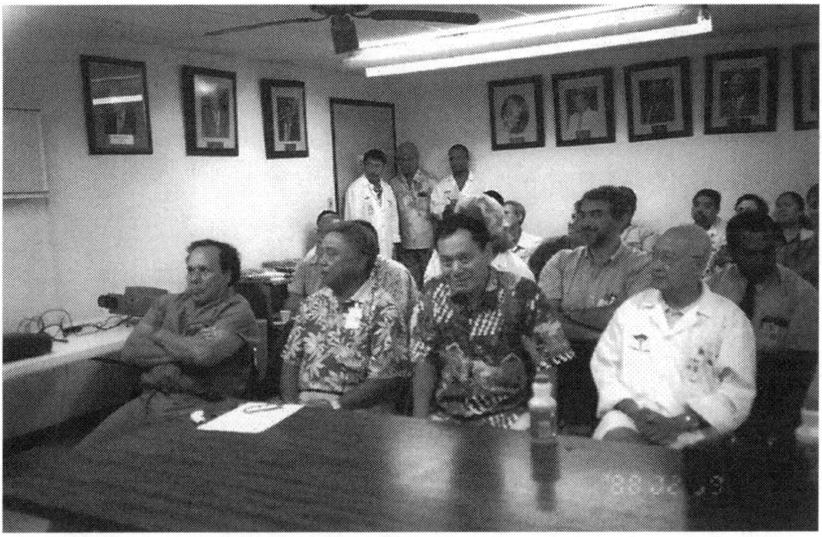

Lecture room at the LBJ Medical Center

Dr. Paopao, far left in scrubs; the author, second from right.

Chapter 3

History of Samoa

HISTORICAL TIMELINE*

1300 BC – The Lapita people once again take to the open seas about this time, pushing east past the Solomon Islands to the Bismarck archipelago and beyond to Vanuatu, Fiji and Samoa. These Southeast Asian peoples had headed south from Taiwan to Papua New Guinea and as far as the main Solomon Islands, where they stopped some 40,000 years ago.

950 AD – Tongans conquer Samoa and rule until *Tuna, Fata`,* and *Savea* drive them from the country. *Malietoa* (brave warrior) becomes a *Matai* title.

1000 AD – *Faiga* becomes *Malietoa.* He abandons cannibalism by not eating his son *Polu.* He gives his granddaughters titles. One becomes *Gato`aitele,* and the other *Tamasoali`i.*

1550 AD – A great woman named *Nafanua* from *Falealupo, Savai`i* is the ruler and gains the *Tafa`ifa* title. The Samoan high chief marries the daughter of the Tongan king. Their daughter, *Salamasina,* is adopted by *So`oa`e,* the widow of

---

*From FamilySearch, "Samoa (Western and American)." © 2021. https://www.familysearch.org/en/wiki/Samoa_(Western_and_American). Reprinted under the Creative Commons Attribution-ShareAlike 4.0 International license. https://creativecommons.org/licenses/by-sa/4.0/legalcode

the high chief of *Atua* district. *Salamasina* also possesses royal Fijian and Tongan blood from her mother.

1700 AD – *Tupua* becomes the progenitor of the *Sa Tupua* family, who has the right to kingship for 100 years.

1722 AD – Dutchman *Jacob Roggeveen* trades in Samoa.

1768 AD – Frenchman *Antoine De Bougainville* trades with Samoans.

1800 AD – White traders begin to settle in Samoa.

1802 AD – *Malietoa Vai`inupo* is appointed king after the death of King *I`amafana.*

1830 AD – *John Williams* of the London Missionary Society brings Christianity to Samoa.

1835 AD – Methodists and London Missionary Society agree that Methodists will proselyte in Tonga and leave Samoa to the London Missionary Society.

1840 AD – *Malietoa Vai`inpo* dies. *Moli Malietoa, Tamasese, Tui-Aj`ana,* and *Mata`afa Tui-Atua* contend for power.

1849 AD – *Willliam T. Pritchard* sets up the first permanent store.

1855 AD – *Goddeffroy and Sons* of Germany establish a store.

1861 AD – *Maliatoa* dies and his sons *Laupepa* and *Talavou* battle over the *Malietoa* title.

1873 AD – Peace is declared between *Laupepa* and *Talavou.* Colonel *A. Steinberger* of the USA helps the Samoans establish a government. *Tupua Pule* declares himself king. Alternating 4-year terms for each king begin.

1875 AD – *Steinberger* becomes premier of *Samoa.*

1880 AD – *Talavou* dies. *Laupepa* becomes king, *Tamasese Sa Tupua* becomes vice-king, and *Mata`afa Sa Tupua* becomes prime minister. They wage a bloody war for power.

1860-89 AD – Samoa exports cotton. Europeans purchase large amounts of land from Samoans.

1889 AD – A devastating hurricane hits. German, British, and American warships sink. *Malieatoa* is crowned king of

Samoa and *Mata'afa* is given a high position. The land commission declares foreign land claims invalid and purchase of land outside Apia forbidden to non-Samoans. *Robert Louis Stevenson* moves to Samoa and he dies 5 years later and is buried on Mt. Vea.

1890 AD – Wars occur between *Malietoa Laupepa* and *Mata`afa.*

1899 AD – *Laupepa*'s son, *Tanumafili* is installed as king by force of foreign powers.

1899 AD – USA, Great Britain and Germany agree to Western Samoa's independence and neutrality. They set up a multi-government. Kingship is abolished in Samoa.

1900 AD – Great Britain Genealogy and Germany cede rights to the islands east of 171 degrees west of Greenwich. Later, a few other islands are added. At present this is unincorporated territory of the United States. Western Samoa becomes a German protectorate and *Heinrich Solf* is governor for ten years. Workers migrate from Micronesia and Melanesia to help on plantations. Eastern Samoa (Tutuila and surrounding islands) become a U.S.A. protectorate.

1903 AD – Over two thousand Chinese laborers are imported to Samoa.

1905 AD – The volcano *Matavanu* on Savai`i erupts and the refugees move to two villages on Upolu.

1910 AD – *Dr. Eric Schultz* is governor of Samoa and the *Malietoa* and *Tupua* families are given titles as counselors to the governor.

1914 AD – Western Samoa is occupied by a New Zealand force during World War I.

1918 AD – A deadly flu epidemic kills one-fifth of the Samoan population (approximately 8,000 people).

1920 AD – New Zealand administers the islands because Germany loses the war.

1920s AD – Schools are built in Sauniatu and Mapusaga.

1923 AD – *Major George Richardson* becomes administrator and dissension between him and Samoans begins.

1929 AD – The Independence movement *(Mau*) becomes a political power.

1939 AD – U.S. Marines establish airfields and a radio station in Eastern Samoa during World War II.

1951 AD – American Samoa administered by the U.S.A. Department of the Interior instead of the Navy.

1954 AD – A Constitutional convention is held to prepare Western Samoa for independence.

1962 AD – Western Samoa becomes an independent country, which renames itself the Independent State of Samoa.

According to legend, Samoa is known as the "Cradle of Polynesia" because Savai'i Island is said to be *Hawaiki*, the Polynesian homeland. Samoan culture is undoubtedly central to Polynesian life, and its styles of music, dance and visual art have gained renown throughout the Pacific islands and the world.

Samoa is the native name of the group of islands in central Polynesia long known as the Navigator Islands. They are situated about 2,600 miles southwest of Honolulu and about 2,000 miles northeast of New Zealand.

The two largest islands—Savai'i and Upolu—plus a few small islands make up Samoa, what used to be known as Western Samoa. The Island of Tutuila and a few smaller islands make up American Samoa.

Even though American Samoa and Samoa are now politically divided, John often reminded me that there was no difference to him—he still had many relatives in (Western) Samoa and the language and customs were the same. Interestingly, the people in American Samoa speak English with an American accent, while those in Samoa do so with a Kiwi accent.

John warned me that when in Pago Pago, American Samoa, if I wanted to call someone in Apia, Samoa, I should be aware that Apia is 25 hours ahead of Pago Pago. As Samoa is a great deal more politically and commercially aligned to New Zealand than America, they decided to keep time with New Zealand instead of with American Samoa.

When I was Pago Pago in 2004, I wanted to check out Apia. Unfortunately, the only flight that day on a small plane from Pago Pago was cancelled. Even though it was just a short distance, the airfare was almost half that of a flight from Honolulu. I was told that there were no passenger ferries between the two cities. This made me conclude that there must not be large numbers of people travelling between them.

It seems that the two Samoas, though not culturally divided, are indeed politically as well as economically divided.

The pre-Western history of American Samoa (formerly Eastern Samoa) is inextricably bound with the history of Samoa (formerly Western Samoa).

The origins of the Samoans are closely studied in modern research about Polynesia in various scientific disciplines such as genetics, linguistics and anthropology. Scientific research is ongoing, although a number of different theories exist, including one proposing that Samoans originated from Austronesian predecessors speaking Oceanic languages during the eastward Lapita expansion period from Southeast Asia and Melanesia between 2,500 and 1,500 BCE. New Zealand scientists have dated remains in Samoa to about 2,900–3,500 years ago. These were found at a Lapita site at Mulifanua and the findings were published in 1974.

Intimate sociocultural and genetic ties were maintained between Samoa, Fiji and Tonga, and archaeological records support oral tradition and native genealogies that indicate inter-island voyaging and intermarriage between pre-colonial Samoans, Fijians and Tongans.

Legends suggest that the Tui Manu'a kings ruled a confederacy of far-flung islands that included Fiji and Tonga as well as smaller western Pacific chiefdoms and Polynesian outliers such as Uvea, Futuna, Tokelau and Tuvalu.

The indigenous political system, the *fa'amatai*, and the culture and customs of *fa'a Sāmoa* ("the Samoan way") originated with two of the most famous early chiefs of Samoa, who were both women and related, Nafanua and Salamasina.

Modern-day Samoa is still united under its two principal royal families: the Sā Malietoa of the ancient Malietoa lineage that defeated the Tongans in the 13th century; and the Sā Tupua, Queen Salamasina's descendants and heirs who ruled Samoa in the centuries that followed her reign.

Within these two principal lineages are the four highest titles of Samoa—the elder titles of *Malietoa* and *Tupua Tamasese* of antiquity, as well as the newer *Mata'afa* and *Tuimalealiifano* titles that rose to prominence in the 19th century wars that preceded the colonial period.

These four titles form the apex of the Samoan *matai* (chief) system as it stands today.

Historically, commerce and exchange routes between western Polynesian societies are well documented. It's speculated that the Tui Manu'a dynasty grew through its success in obtaining control over the oceanic trade of goods such as finely woven ceremonial mats, whale ivory objects, obsidian and basalt tools, red feathers and seashells reserved for royalty.

Early Western contact with Samoa began in the early 18th century. Jacob Roggeveen, a Dutchman, was the first known non-Polynesian to sight the Samoan islands in 1722. Further European included a battle between French explorers and the islanders in Tutuila, during which the Samoans gained a reputation for ferocity. This was followed by French explorer Louis-Antoine de Bougainville, who named them the Navigator Islands in 1768.

Early 19th century Rarotongan missionaries to the Samoan islands were followed by a group of Western missionaries led by John Williams of the (Congregationalist) London Missionary Society in the 1830s, officially bringing Christianity to Samoa. At that time, whaler and traders also began arriving.

The Samoas in the 1800s

Visits by American trading and whaling vessels were important in the early economic development of Samoa.

The Salem brig *Roscoe*, arriving in October 1821, was the first American trading vessel known to have visited. The *Maro* of Nantucket, in 1824, was the first recorded United States whaler at Samoa. The whalers came for fresh drinking water, firewood and provisions, and later they recruited local men to serve as crewmen on their ships. The last recorded whaler visitor was the *Governor Morton* in 1870.

In 1872, the high chief of the tribes of the eastern Samoan islands gave America permission to establish a naval base in exchange for military protection. In 1878, the U.S. Navy built a coaling station on Pago Pago Bay for its Pacific Squadron and appointed a local Secretary.

Britain also sent troops to protect British business enterprise, harbor rights and consulate office. This was followed by an eight-year civil war, during which each of the three powers supplied arms, training and in some cases combat troops to the warring Samoan parties. The Samoan crisis came to a critical juncture in March 1889 when all three colonial contenders sent warships into Apia harbor, and a larger-scale war seemed imminent. A massive storm on March 15, 1889 damaged or destroyed the warships, ending the military conflict.

The Second Samoan Civil War reached a head in 1898 when Germany, Britain and the United States were locked in dispute over who should control the Samoan Islands. The Siege of Apia occurred in March 1899. Samoan forces loyal to Prince Tanu were besieged by a larger force of Samoan rebels loyal to Mata'afa Iosefo. Supporting Prince Tanu were landing parties from four British and American warships. After several days of fighting, the Samoan rebels were finally defeated.

American Samoa is the result of the Second Samoan Civil War and an agreement made between Germany, the United States and Britain in the Tripartite Convention of 1899. The international rivalries were settled by the 1899 Treaty of Berlin, in which Germany and the U.S. divided the Samoan archipelago. Several chiefs of the island of Tutuila swore allegiance and ceded the island to the United States in the Treaty of Cession of Tutuila of 1900. The eastern Samoan islands became territories of the United States and later became known as American Samoa.

The Samoas in the 1900s

The German Empire governed the western part of the Samoan archipelago from 1900 to 1914. Wilhelm Solf was appointed the colony's first governor. In 1908, when the non-violent Mau a Pule Resistance Movement arose, Solf banished the Mau leader Lauaki Namulau'ulu Mamoe to Saipan in the German Northern Mariana Islands.

In the first month of World War I, on August 29, 1914, troops of the New Zealand Expeditionary Force landed unopposed on Upolu and seized control from the German authorities, following a request by Great Britain.

After World War I, the Mau Movement in Western Samoa (then a New Zealand protectorate) began.

The Mau Movement was a non-violent movement for Samoan independence from colonial rule during the first half of the 20th century. Mau means *resolute* or *resolved*, also denoting *firm strength* in Samoan. The motto for the Mau was *Samoa mo Samoa* (Samoa for the Samoans).

The movement had its beginnings on the island of Savai'i with the Mau a Pule Resistance in the early 1900s, with widespread support throughout the country by the late 1920s. As the movement grew, leadership came under the country's chiefly elite, the customary matai leaders entrenched in Samoan tradition and *fa'a Sāmoa*. The Mau included women who supported the national organization through leadership and organization as well as taking part in marches. Supporters wore a Mau uniform of a navy blue lavalava (a square of cloth tied at the waist, similar to a wraparound skirt) with a white stripe, which was later banned by the colonial administration.

The Mau movement culminated on December 28, 1929 in the streets of the capital Apia, when New Zealand military police fired on a procession that was attempting to prevent the arrest of one of its members. The day became known as Black Saturday. Up to 11 Samoans were killed, including a Mau leader and one of the paramount chiefs of Samoa, Tupua Tamasese Lealofi III, with many others wounded. One New Zealand constable was clubbed to death by protesters following the outbreak of hostilities.

The Mau Movement's efforts would ultimately result in the political independence of Samoa in 1962.

After World War I, there was a corresponding American Samoa Mau Movement, led by Samuel Sailele Ripley, a World War I veteran from Leone village. In 1921, 17 chiefs of the American Samoa Mau were arrested and imprisoned under hard labor.

During World War II, U.S. Marines in American Samoa outnumbered the local population, having a huge cultural influence. Young Samoan men from the age of 14 and above were combat trained by U.S. military personnel. As in World War

I, American Samoans served in World War II as combatants, medical personnel, code personnel, ship repairmen, etc.

After WWII, a U.S. Department of Interior-sponsored attempt to incorporate American Samoa was made, but it was defeated in Congress, primarily through the efforts of American Samoan chiefs led by Tuiasosopo Mariota. These chiefs' efforts led to the creation of a local legislature, the American Samoa *Fono,* which meets in the village of Fagatogo, the territory's capital.

In time, the Navy-appointed governor was replaced by a locally elected one. American Samoa is self-governing under a constitution that became effective on July 1, 1967. In spite of this, the islands have been reluctant to separate from the U.S. in any manner.

Samoa, now officially the Independent State of Samoa and until 1997 known as Western Samoa, is a unitary parliamentary democracy with 11 administrative divisions.

The sovereign state is a member of the Commonwealth of Nations as a Commonwealth republic. Western Samoa was admitted to the United Nations on December 15, 1976.

Chapter 4
Pago Pago

MY FIRST IMPRESSION OF THE ISLAND OF TUTUILA was that it was probably how Hawaii looked a hundred years ago, when there were no crowds, no high rises and not much noise.

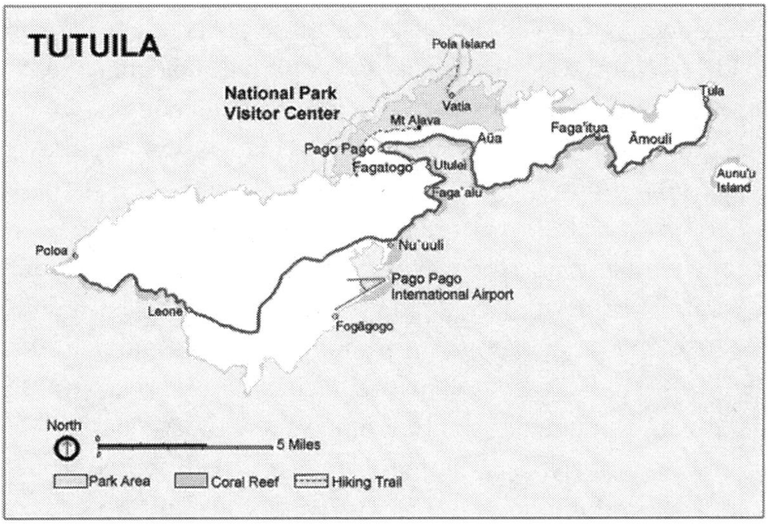

American Samoa

There didn't seem to be a lot of air traffic at the Tafuna International Airport, except for flights to and from Hawaii, neighboring islands and the independent country of (Western) Samoa. The small terminal was in the process of expanding, and taxis were readily available when we exited the building.

The capital city of American Samoa, Pago Pago (pronounced Pango Pango), sits at the western end of a bay on the island, approximately 16 miles from the airport. Remote and stunningly beautiful, the lush, tropical location made me think this was how paradise must look.

Our group checked into the Tradewinds Hotel—I was told it was the newest and nicest hotel in town. A group of official-looking people, five men and two women, who had been on the same flight with us, were also checking in. We soon learned that these were FBI and IRS agents sent to investigate the pervasive corruption in the territory.

It seemed that the governor himself was the main target, going down to different levels and departments. We learned that the LBJ hospital was chronically lacking multiple drugs, and for a period of time there was no morphine or even codeine for pain. Some critics claimed that the shortage was because of corruption.

It just happened to be election time for American Samoa, and banners and posters were everywhere. One I found notable for its lack of originality read, "Yes, We Can," a sentiment I'd seen so many times before, in so many countries and in different languages—most recently in the Mexican election, with their rally cry of "Sí, se puede'" and in Malaysia with, "Ya kita boleh."

It was unlikely that the federal government would clean up all the corruption because this was part of the culture. I learned that one of the reasons few Samoans own and run stores is because their relatives and friends would think nothing of simply taking what they wanted without paying, since it was their custom to share.

The practice extended to jobs as well. If you're Samoan, you're supposed to take care of your family and relatives. If you're the head of a department, you would make sure your nephews and nieces got the first crack at any job openings.

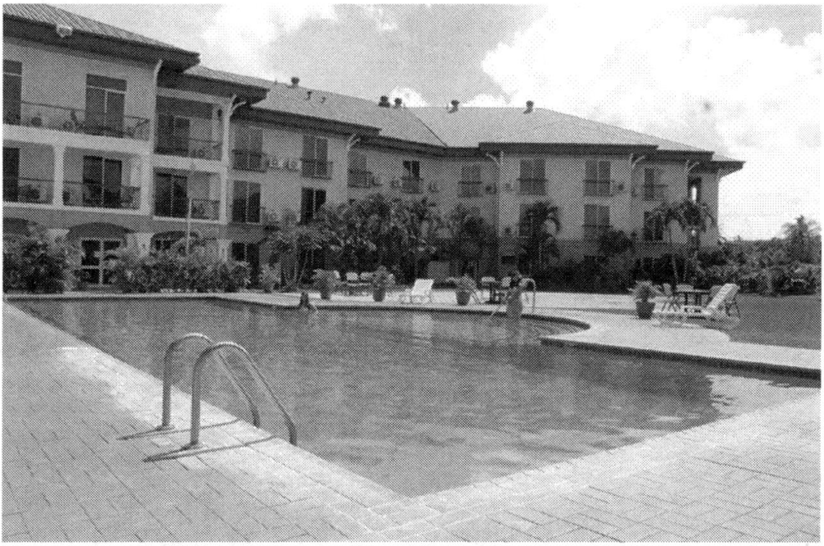

The Tradewinds Hotel, the nicest in Pago Pago in 2004.

Housed in the historic Post Office and Navy Commissary buildings was the Jean P. Haydon Museum in Fagatogo, of which John's sister Sao was the administrator. It was named after the wife of the founder, who collected many of the artifacts now on display. Sao was kind enough to give us a special tour and each a set of four coffee mugs with Samoan floral patterns.

The museum showcased Samoan history, culture and nature. It featured many cultural artifacts such as clothing, art, weaponry, pottery and tattooing. There were also artifacts from WWII. Exhibits about the island itself, including the types of plants and animals, were also on display. I learned that the area was prone to hurricanes, earthquakes and tsunamis.

Five years after our visit, on September 29, 2009, Pago Pago was inundated by a tsunami generated by an undersea earthquake of magnitude 8.3, centered some 120 miles (190 km) to the south in the Pacific Ocean. The tsunami caused extensive damage in the city and throughout the Samoan archipelago, resulting in scores of deaths and the destruction of many villages.

While we were there, Sao served us kava, the national drink made from the roots of a native plant. It was a great place to learn about the island and become acquainted with the local culture before venturing out to other destinations.

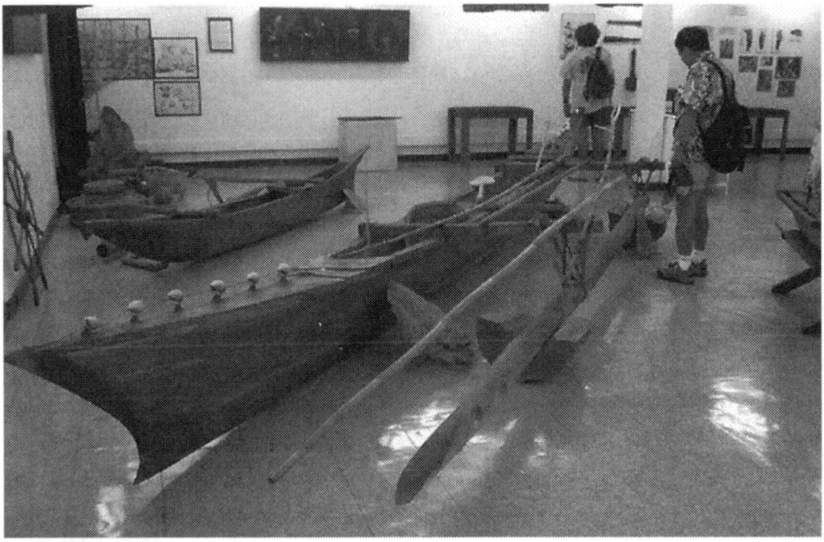

The Museum
Ancient canoes and weapons.

One Saturday, we climbed Mount Alava. At almost 500 meters above sea level, it had sweeping views of Pago Pago harbor. John told us this was an excellent place to check out the region's ecosystem, which included fruit bats, geckos and wild dogs.

There were also many fantastic beaches on the island. Snorkeling was wonderful around the coral reef that fringes the island, home to hundreds of species of coral and nearly one thousand different kinds of fish. I learned that Whitetip reef sharks, sea turtles, porpoises, giant clams and barracudas, among other marine creatures, lived in the surrounding waters.

As I walked along the beach road one afternoon, I noticed many individual fishermen selling their catch. One was selling a large spiny lobster that weighed over ten pounds for only $10 U.S. (the currency in American Samoa was of course the U.S. dollar).

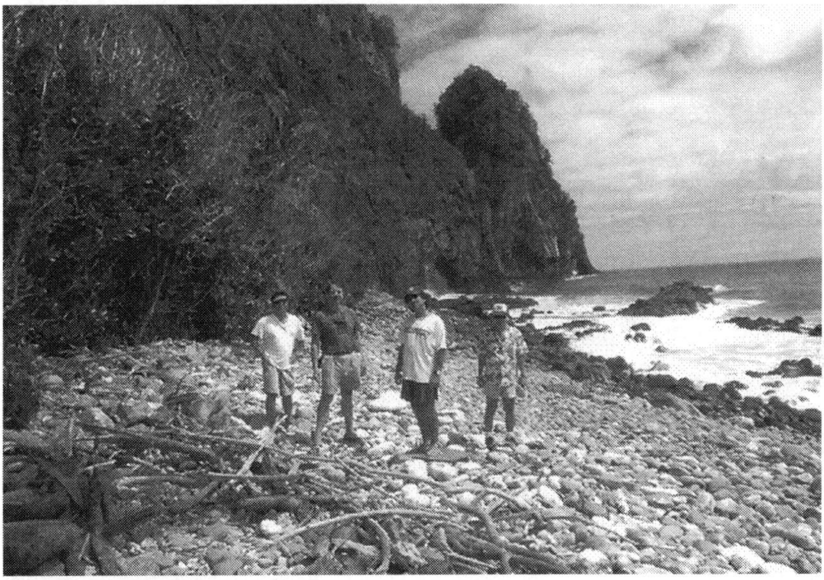

On a beach near Pago Pago
From left: Drs. Tom Namiki, Douglas Johnson, Steve Garon and the author.

Exploring along the Route 1 ocean road, we stopped by the Sadie Thompson Inn, whose namesake was made famous by W. Somerset Maugham in the short story "Rain" after the writer's stay there.

Pago Plaza was a hub for small stores selling handicrafts, while Fagatogo Square Shopping Center had ethnic restaurants and larger stores where one could find American-style clothing as well as Samoan fashions. The traditional *puletasi* dresses with the typical Samoan designs were abundantly available. Snorkeling and swim supplies were sold in several shops.

Near the dock at the harbor and on the main street, locals sold handmade crafts such as beautiful mats and baskets made from coconut leaves and other fibers.

Local growers came to sell their bananas, coconuts, breadfruit and other fresh produce at the market near the bus station at the end of Fagatogo village. The big market day was Saturday as they were closed on Sunday. Most Samoans go to church on Sunday.

The two tuna canneries employed most workers in the private sector. They were in the mile-long industrial complex on the north coast of the harbor. Nearest to Pago Pago was Starkist. The other was COS Packing. John told me that most of the workers at the canneries were from Western Samoa.

Tutuila's villages have preserved *fa'a Sāmoa,* the Samoan way, so residents have a strong sense of tradition and observe many of the customs that began with their ancestors 3,000 years ago. Traditional meals are eaten while seated on the floor. Businesses are closed on Sundays. Nearly all of the population primarily speaks Samoan, despite the predominance of English.

I thoroughly enjoyed my time on Tutuila. It was a beautiful island and Pago Pago was a charming town. I left thinking that one could easily fall in love with that sort of lifestyle.

Chapter 5
The Lyndon B. Johnson Tropical Medical Center

ALL OF OUR WORK WAS DONE at the Lyndon B. Johnson Tropical Medical Center, the only hospital in American Samoa, located in the Faga'alu Valley, Maoputasi County.

Built in 1968 on nearly 20 acres, the hospital has been ranked among the best hospitals in the Pacific Ocean. It's home to an emergency room and there are doctors on duty at all hours. It is a 150-bed facility and includes most of the medical and surgical departments, with the exception of neurosurgery and some subspecialties.

The LBJ Tropical Medical Center had become familiar to me through ophthalmology journals, because for years, whenever I opened my eye journals, LBJ would be advertising for an ophthalmologist. Later I learned that because of the remote location and low pay, the medical center had trouble keeping a good ophthalmologist—or any ophthalmologist for that matter. Each new ophthalmologist simply kicked the can further down the road. Many cataracts needed surgery but few were done. Diabetic patients with retinopathy went untreated.

As LBJ was administered by the U.S. Public Health Service, there was a lot of red tape regarding employment. I learned that, in the past, almost all the ophthalmologists who served at LBJ were older practitioners from the U.S. who had retired from their own private practices and were looking for an adventure, no longer interested in working hard.

In spite of this, the medical center has maintained a good reputation over the years. A 1971 study found that the hospital services offered at LBJ compared favorably with services offered at similar-sized facilities in the continental U.S. The Samoan government began sending more medical students for training, mostly to Fiji with a few in the U.S, and nurses for RN training in Hawaii. New programs in the 1970s offered maternal and child health education, chronic and communicable disease control, filariasis control, and mental health services.

In addition, renal dialysis equipment arrived and a special unit was organized. It soon became one of the most valuable additions to local healing services as kidney disease increased because of the extremely high incidence of diabetes. I was told that as many as 50% of the residents in America Samoa had diabetes. The incidence of obesity and hypertension were high as well, both of which contribute to renal failure.

Prior to 1982, medical services provided at LBJ were free to local residents. Even with subsidies from the U.S. Department of the Interior, and several million from Medicare and Medicaid, it was still running a deficit.

Another problem was that the hospital had trouble hiring and keeping U.S.-trained physicians. Most of the physicians at LBJ were trained in Fiji and some in Papua New Guinea. Because the medical center was administered by the U.S. government, it would only pay for services provided by a U.S.-licensed physician.

When we arrived in 2004, I learned that the only U.S.-trained physician on staff was being investigated by the U.S. government for fraud, because of almost all the payments were going to him (in his name, on behalf of the hospital), which amounted to several million dollars. In order for the medical center to get paid by Medicare for services provided by the physicians trained in Fiji and Solomon Islands, all charges had to be signed by the U.S.-trained physician. The investigation was launched after some bureaucrats at Medicare decided that it was physically impossible for one physician to have provided so much service to so many patients.

This issue was resolved after the medical center explained that this doctor was able to charge so much to Medicare and Medicaid because he was the overseer of all the other physicians.

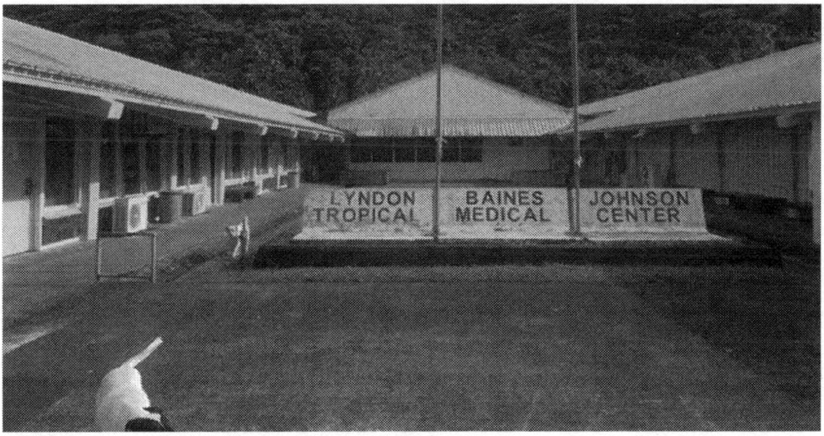

The LBJ Medical Center in Pago Pago.

On Monday, a conference was held at the hospital at noon, during which I gave a lecture on the treatment of diabetic retinopathy. With the incidence of diabetes among the residents so high, some of the patients had gone blind from untreated diabetic retinopathy, while others had undergone amputations of feet and legs.

As most physicians went through medical school without having taken a rotation in ophthalmology, some of them had little knowledge of what could be done for the retinopathy of these diabetic patients. My lecture went over how laser treatment was done. The treatment was amazingly simple and the success rate was almost 100%. Many of the physicians present at the lecture that day confided to me later that it was the first time they truly understood how the laser treatment worked and they were amazed that it was so simple for the patient, as it required no cutting and usually no anesthesia, and most patients tolerated the procedure very well.

The ophthalmologist in charge at the LBJ Medical Center was Dr. Khin Oo, a Burmese native who was recruited from New Zealand. After leaving Yangon, the capital of Burma, he and his wife were able to land in New Zealand. He worked in a hospital for a time but was never able to get licensed for private practice. When LBJ was again looking for an ophthalmologist, he applied and got the job, and had been there for over five years when I met him.

Dr. Oo was proud of what he had done for the department. He was a meticulous man and had all the patients with diabetes in a registry.

During my visit, I did a number of laser treatments for diabetic retinopathy. I had brought along my own laser as I usually did when I went on a medical mission. Dr. Oo was happy to talk to another ophthalmologist, as he felt very isolated on the island.

The following day, a forty-year-old man showed up at the clinic complaining that he couldn't see out of his right eye. Over the weekend, this man, a worker at the tuna cannery, was drinking beer with several of his friends and they got into a fight. He was punched in the face.

That evening, he saw numerous black spots as well as flashing lights. The following morning, the eye was blind and he decided to come to the clinic.

Dr. Oo examined him and noted a detached retina. He asked me if I would do the surgery as he hadn't been trained for it, which I was happy to do.

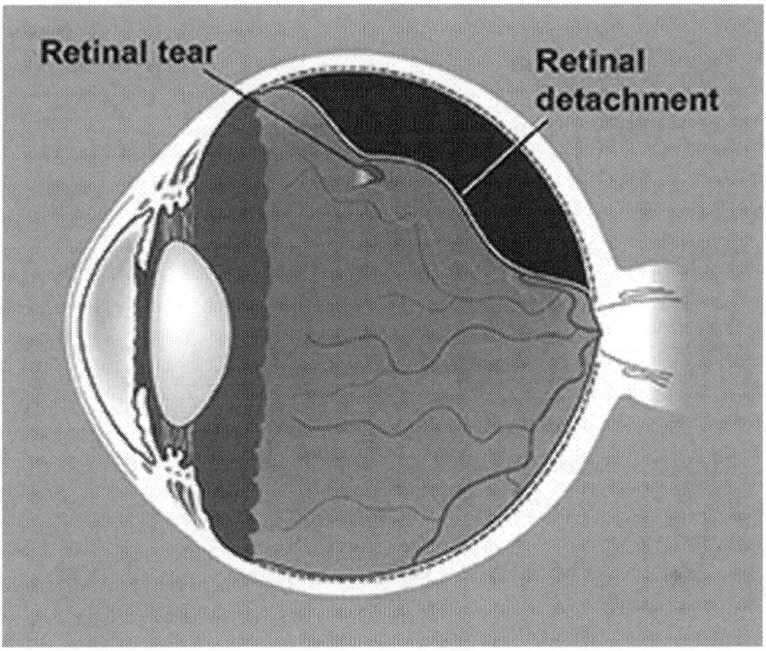

A detached retina with a retinal tear

I'd brought along the basic supplies and instrument for such a surgery. It was done with local anesthesia and took less than an hour. The hospital's cryo machine wasn't working, so I was glad I had my laser machine. I would normally use the cryo machine to seal a retinal tear during such a surgery, but I was able to seal it with the laser instead.

When we saw the patient the following day, his retina was fully attached and he was able to see out of the eye again.

Dr. Oo also presented me with some patients that he wanted a second opinion on. Some of them who suffered from diabetic retinopathy were too advanced to benefit from the laser treatment, and unfortunately they were already almost totally blind.

I found Dr. Oo to be a very intelligent man and a skillful cataract surgeon. I'd examined some of his cataract surgery patients and they all seemed to have good vision. None of them had any complications.

By 4 pm on Thursday, we were caught up with our patients at the clinic, and Dr. Oo decided to give me a tour of Pago Pago. We went to the main public market. All sorts of fruits, vegetables and roots such as taro were on sale. Dr. Oo pointed out some of the green vegetables he and his wife liked, vegetables that reminded them of home. I was impressed with the variety of taro I saw. They were gigantic, each over two feet long and weighing over 20 pounds, whereas the taro found in Hawaii usually measured just over half a foot and weighed less than five pounds.

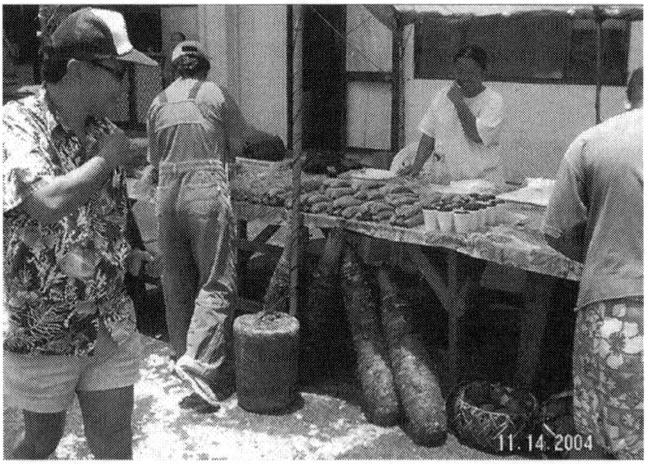

Checking out the local market. Note the gigantic taro under the vendor's table. Each taro can weigh 20 to 30 lbs.

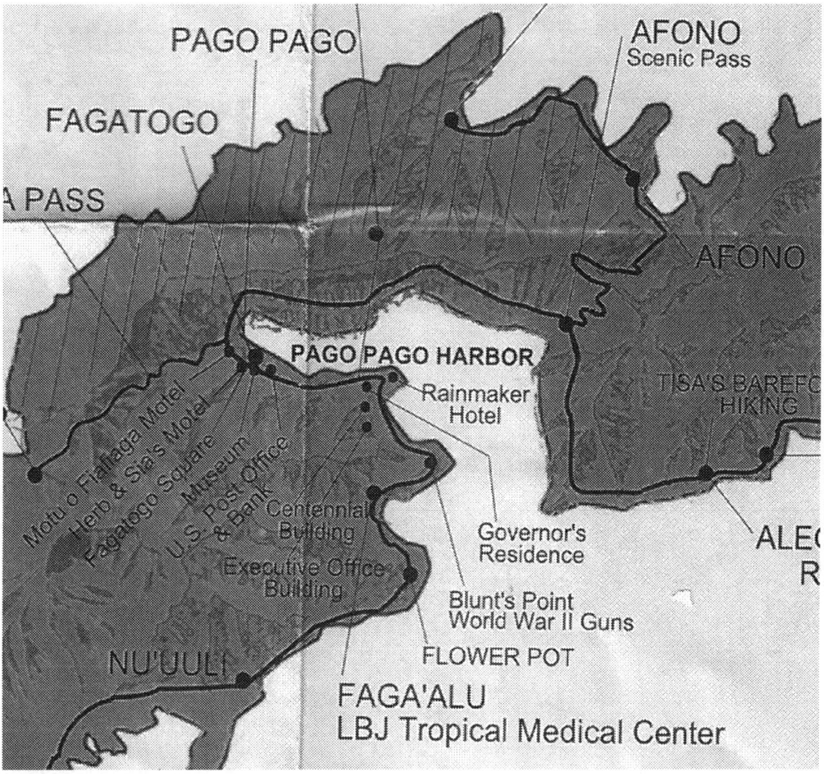

Major landmarks of Pago Pago

We stopped by a food stand at the market where a Chinese couple was selling stir-fried noodles. We each ordered a plate of yellow egg noodles with shrimp and calamari. I learned that the couple had emigrated from Hong Kong recently and their goal was to settle in California eventually, after establishing residency in American Samoa. The food stand seemed popular, with people standing in line to order their noodles.

Dr. Oo seemed pleased with his work at LBJ but lamented that it was difficult to train local doctors. "Two years ago, we sent a very intelligent local woman to get additional training in Sydney," he said. "She had graduated from the medical school in Fiji, which was a respected institution, and spent two years at the Pacific Eye Institute to train as an ophthalmologist. But after a few months in Sydney she got pregnant and returned home, and decided that she wasn't going to work as a doctor after all, since her husband had a good job. It was such a waste of resources.

"Then there's this young doc I've been trying to train to take over my job when I leave in a few years. He seems distracted a lot of the time. Just last week, over the weekend, he treated a man from a remote village with a corneal ulcer. He and I have treated many of these before. I always stressed to him that if you suspect infection on the cornea, never patch the eye because the patching would only encourage the infection. So, what did he do? He patched the eye and when we saw the patient on Monday, the infection had gotten worse. The poor patient almost lost his eye. I was so disappointed with him because it seems like such a simple thing, and yet he couldn't do it correctly," he lamented.

Dr. Oo seemed like a deep thinker and was philosophical about life. He was sad about the conditions in Burma. "James, you know, before World War II, Burma was so much more advanced than countries like Thailand and Malaysia. We had excellent universities. The medical school I went to was known as the Edinburgh of the Far East, because many of the professors were from Edinburgh University and it had very high standards. Graduates could practice anywhere in the world. One of my cousins went to Hong Kong and became a professor at the University of Hong Kong Medical School. Now all the universities are run-down and the professors live like paupers. Anyone who could leave has left," he sighed.

After we finished our noodles and left the market, Dr. Oo drove me around and showed me more landmarks on the island. He dropped me off at my hotel just as the golden tropical sun was setting into the horizon, and as it set, just before disappearing, I was able to see a green flash for a second.

The green flash is an optical phenomenon that you can see shortly after sunset or before sunrise. It happens when the sun is almost entirely below the horizon, with the barest edge visible. For a second or two, that upper rim of the sun will appear green in color.

Chapter 6
A Samoan Feast

AFTER WORKING VERY HARD, the first week ended well for all of us. That Friday afternoon, we were invited to a village for a Samoan feast. It was obvious that John, the grandson of a chief, was a popular and respected fellow in American Samoa.

We arrived at the village around 5 pm. Samoa is full of tall mountains and beautiful beaches, and most villages aren't far from the water. This beach was near the village where John grew up.

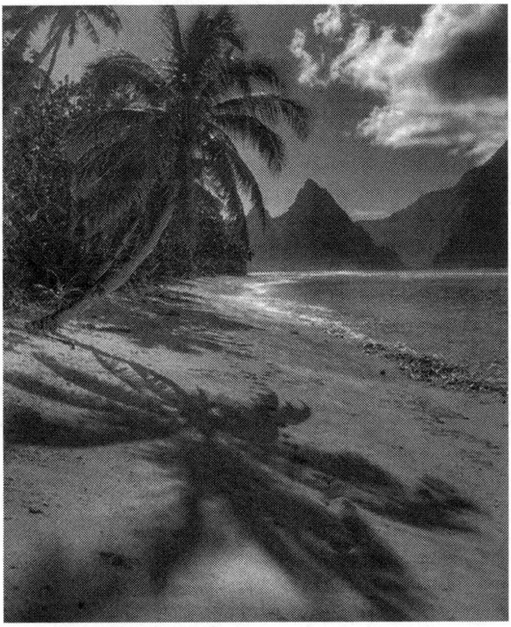

Feast by the beach

A *fale tele*, or big house, is used by villagers as a meeting house for chiefs, for family gatherings and for ceremonies such as weddings and funerals. It's usually situated in a prominent location within the village.

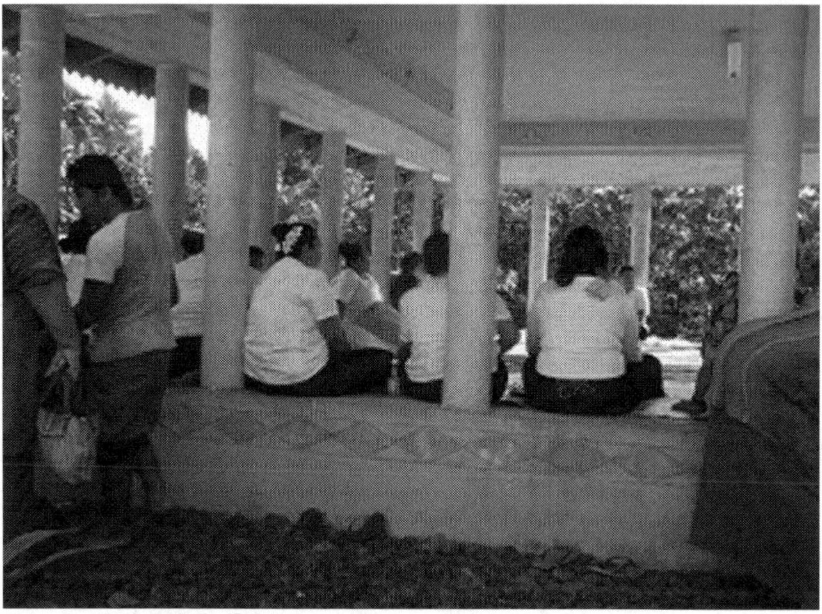

Guests sitting in a *fale*

The occasion was John's homecoming. The roasting pit, or the *umu,* had been prepared early in the morning. The roast pig was the center of attention. It took hours of preparation to get the pig ready for the perfect *umu*. The 200-lb. pig had to be cleaned thoroughly and seasoned with sea salt. Then it was stuffed with leaves, roots and vegetable that had been soaked in coconut milk.

The pig was laid on a bed of banana leaves, then surrounded by hot rocks. The cooks made sure that the skin wasn't in direct contact with the hot rocks, which would burn it. Instead, it was protected by several layers of banana leaves.

It took almost the whole day to cook the pig.

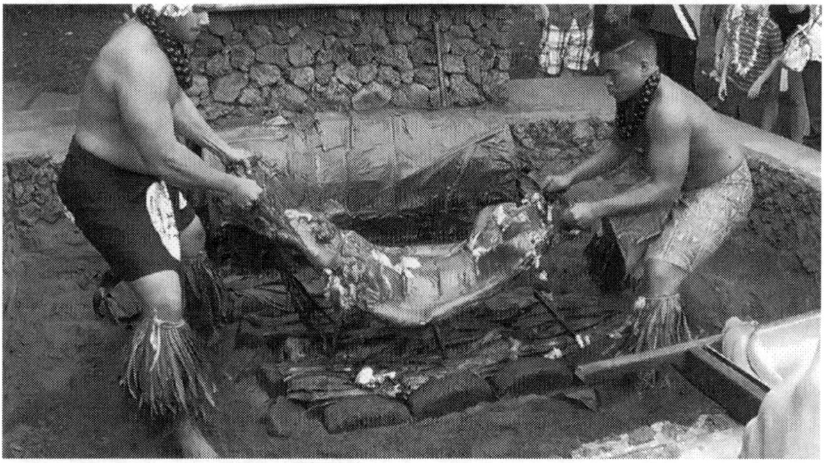

Roast a pig in the roasting pit, the *umu*

The Samoan Umu Feast is about reconnecting in a family-friendly atmosphere, sharing travel adventure stories and meeting new friends. The local beer called Vailima, meaning Five Rivers, was served and flowed freely. At 6 pm, as the sun was setting, the ceremony began.

The top village chief spoke briefly, and then the speaking-chief performed a ceremony filled with chants followed by a speech in Samoan, which I was told was about John's achievements.

John was asked to give a speech, which he did with grace, thanking his elders and family who made it possible to be where he was.

Then the crew went about uncovering the roasted pig. As the bananas leaves were removed, the aroma of the roasted pork permeated the air. The band played a fast tune as the crew carried the pig to the center of the *fale*.

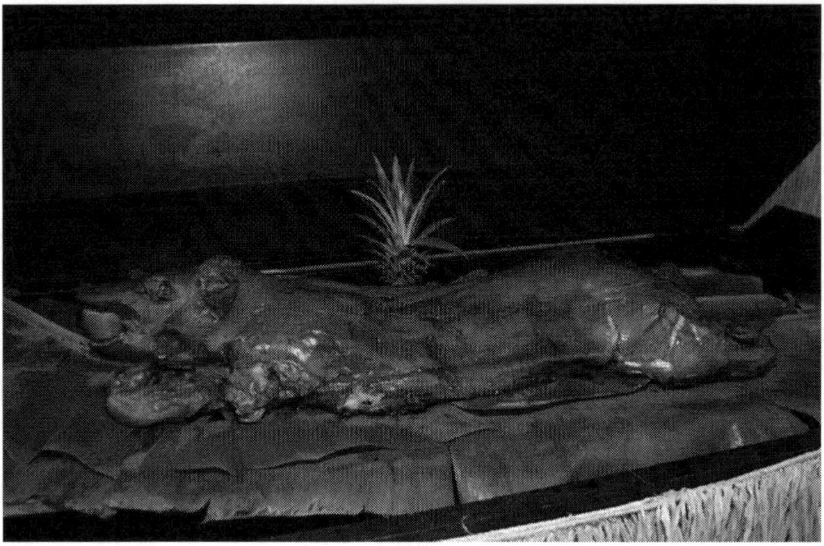

The Roast Pig

Samoa is home to some of the most friendly, hospitable and generous people in the world. Like many cultures, family ties are refreshed and renewed through the sharing of food. Every major life event is marked with a feast—John's homecoming in our case. It's the only meal of the day, with people waking up in the wee hours of the morning to start cooking. Samoan people love to joke around, sing and dance and are serious about only three things in life: God, family and food. As the villagers prepared the feast, gaiety was in the air. People were laughing and singing.

In addition to the roast pig, other items served were roast chicken, vegetable soups, fresh fish wrapped in banana leaves and barbequed, and the Samoan ceviche called *oka*—raw fish marinated in coconut cream served with cucumber, tomato, lime and cilantro.

Many of the dishes were cooked with coconut, such as coconut cream taro, coconut cream yams and coconut cream potatoes. I noticed that Samoan cooking is quite versatile, and the ingredients are actually quite flexible, adaptable to any local produce or meats.

One of the dishes seemed familiar to me, which they called *sapasui* (chop suey), a recipe influenced by the many Chinese who had settled in Samoa. One of my favorite dishes there was the mango-spiced chicken.

Another of my favorite Samoan dishes was one John used to cook whenever I visited him, called *palusami*—spinach or taro leaves cooked with coconut milk and sometimes with corned beef from New Zealand. The taro leaves can be added to soups, stews and casseroles, making them a versatile vegetable. They can also be cooked and eaten plain, similar to other leafy greens like spinach and kale. I was told that it's important to cook them sufficiently to reduce their oxalate content.

Music always accompanied such a feast. On this occasion, there was a band of five young men playing popular Samoan music as others sang along. As we were the guests of honor, we were invited to eat with the elders in the village. The grandparents ate first, then the parents, followed by small children. The young people helped with the cooking and other chores, such as scraping taro or grating coconut meat for coconut milk. They were also responsible for preparing the *apa fafano*, a bowl of warm, soapy water for handwashing and providing a towel for drying.

I noticed that once an elder had finished eating, the younger people would clear their dishes, bring them the *apa fafano* and towel, then offer a hot beverage.

When an elder left the table, the younger generation would clear and reset the vacated spot for the next person in the hierarchy. Only after all the elders had eaten was it acceptable for the rest to dish themselves a plate of what was left of the day's delicacies.

And then it was cleanup, again done by the younger generation.

A young woman, a primary school teacher from the village, explained to me that if the home you're meeting in is yours, never bang pots and pans around or clank the utensils or dishes while you wash and dry them. In Samoan culture, this is a signal that a guest in the home is unwanted. It will cause hurt feelings amongst your guests and could even lead to a not-so-nice retaliation from them.

She told me that her aunt used to call out to her, "E i ai se mea e ke le malie i ai?" ("Is there something you're not happy about?") whenever she accidentally dropped a pot or was making more noise than usual.

Samoan society is clearly well structured. When Westerners first appeared on the scene, they thought the Samoans were barbarians. Later they found out that it was a structured society with a system similar to a democracy. War could not be easily started, and could only be waged after being agreed upon by a majority of chiefs.

I could understand why the Samoans were so proud of their heritage, because in spite of Western influences for hundreds of years, they managed to retain their customs, language and traditions, and have been very successful in keeping the land to themselves, as it's been written into law that only Samoans can hold titles to the land.

Even among Samoans, an individual doesn't hold a land title. Only the village owns the land. If a family needs a plot of land to build a house, the village chiefs will decide. I learned that even a village chief cannot sell the land.

After the feast, I talked and visited with as many people as I could. It was such an honor to be a guest among the villagers. It was obvious that the Samoans treated their guests of honor with great respect. After a couple of Vailima and feeling less inhibited, I invited the friendly school teacher to dance. Then someone invited me to dance. The Samoans truly knew how to throw a party. Everyone was laughing and many were singing along. It was a joyous occasion for their native son to come home for a visit. They were so very proud of John.

By midnight, the crowed slowly drifted away. I will always remember the occasion and my experience of the incomparable Samoan hospitality.

Chapter 7

A Funeral

JOHN USED TO TELL ME STORIES about being afraid of ghosts in the village. Unlike America, after the sun set, the village went dark in most places. As a young boy, he was afraid to go out at night because of the people buried in front of the houses.

What puzzled and scared John as a child was that his relatives would talk to the buried people as if they were alive. He heard stories from other boys about how they had seen ghosts and that the dead people would sometimes venture out of their graves to visit the living. It would send chills down John's spine.

On a Saturday, while most of the group was playing golf, I decided to witness a funeral in a village not far from where John grew up. A respected member of the village had died.

Traditional funerals in Samoa last for several days, with events taking place each day. I attended the last day, when the service for the community was conducted, as well as the burial.

Around 9 am, we gathered in an open area where the women's organization (comprised of women from the village and family members) began a processional to the main *fale* where the casket was sitting. They held yards and yards of fabric, which they carried up the stairs and placed around the casket area. The first fabric was white.

After fabric was distributed to the visitors, more gifts were given. Fine mats—an important part of Samoan culture—were also handed out. Gifts were exchanged between the village leaders of the deceased and the village leaders of his wife.

Food was an important part of the ceremony, and containers of chicken, sausage and fish were also distributed among the mourners.

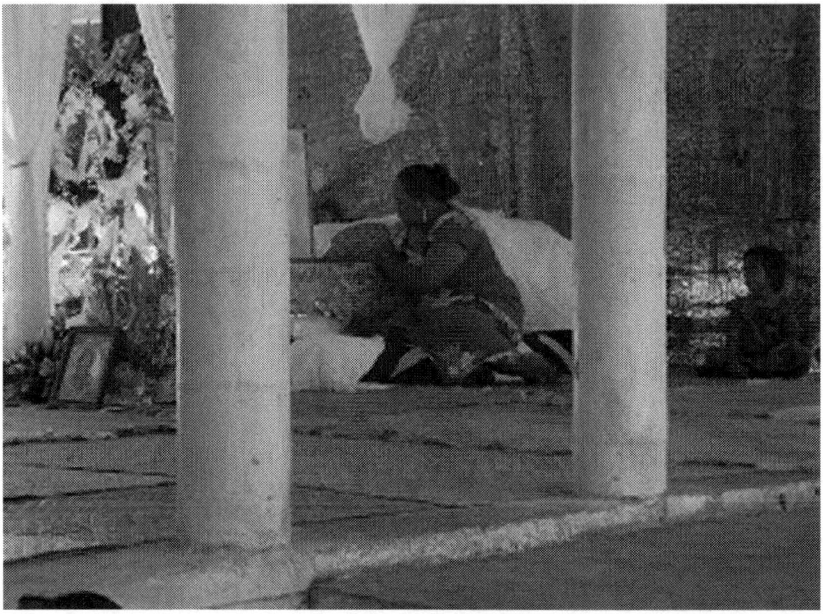

The deceased in a casket for viewing by friends and relatives.

Samoan Death Ceremony

Death never really happens in Samoa, in the sense that the deceased are never treated as though they're gone. They're usually buried in the family's front yard and are talked to often. For Samoans, conversing with those who have passed on is the epitome of their spiritual relationship. Death, in Samoan tradition, is considered God's will. It was traditionally believed that Samoans should die at home; otherwise, one's spirit might cause problems for the family. Before the advancement of mortuary science, the deceased was buried the day after death. Now, it's common to delay funerals for overseas loved ones to arrive.

The talking chief (*tulafale*) is the designated storyteller and funeral leader who has the responsibility of notifying family and friends about the death. Once the appropriate people have been notified, the *matai* (chief) and *tulafale* perform an important ceremony called *saofa'i*, which brings the family together. There may be other high-ranking community members in attendance as well. This meeting is highly important because it's when decisions about the deceased's passing and the funeral are made, and the chief delegates roles and responsibilities to each member of the group.

During the week prior to the funeral, friends, co-workers, extended family and church members visit the immediate family to deliver gifts and show their respect. There are strict rules around these offerings. The talking chief receives the gifts and thanks those who brought them on behalf of the family, and then gives back half of what was given. All gifts are recorded in a notebook and kept by the person assigned to the accounting job.

On the day of the funeral, guests give the grieving family monetary gifts or hand-woven mats in a ceremonial exchange called *fa'alavelave*. As in the pre-funeral rituals, they also might bring boxes of corned beef, canned chicken or tuna.

Appropriate dress for funerals is a *lavalava* (skirt-like wrap), white shirt, tie, jacket and leather sandals for men, and a *pulu tasi* (muumuu) for women.

The service lasts about an hour and a half. The Moomooga Samoan funeral song is sung to say goodbye to the departed. Flowers and food are everywhere in and around the *fale*, and the casket is left open for the viewing.

There is also an *ava* ceremony, sometimes called *kava*, in which a ceremonial drink made from the roots of a pepper plant is served to recognize the event that has occurred.

The mourning period typically lasts about two weeks.

The custom of locating graves beside houses is a unique one. Almost every village house, as well as many in town, has a grave or two nearby.

A chief is more likely to be buried in a conspicuous tomb at the front of the house, while other family members might be buried less conspicuously beside or even behind the house. According to old custom (now rarely observed), if a woman died while living in her husband's village, she was, if possible, returned for burial in her own village. There no longer seems to be a consensus about what the customary rules are for wives and mothers. Each family does as it prefers and common practices are gradually evolving into new customs.

Nowadays, families often inter their parents side by side near the family home. Many graves in both rural and urban areas are incorporated into the structure of the house. For example, one family decided to bury their father, a village *matai*, under a marble-faced tomb on the front veranda of their house. When their mother died, she was buried beside him under a matching tomb. Later, the children of this couple extended the house, and the tombs are now located in the furnished, air-conditioned front room of their house where the family meets for evening prayers.

I learned of another case in which a family who lost their son in a car accident decided to inter him under the house, and his tomb was constructed within what had once been his bedroom.

Graves located beside or in front of houses are built in many styles; they might be enclosed by decorative wrought iron fences or, in an increasingly common practice, enclosed in small houses.

Years ago, headstones were imported; now they can be commissioned locally. Many of these headstones are elaborate and feature photographs of the deceased, decorative urns and statues of angels.

Different cultures treat death of their loved ones differently. I'd never heard of graves beside or in front of houses before I went to American Samoa, and I must admit that it's one of the most surprising customs I've ever encountered.

I found it interesting that, unlike most cultures, Samoan's don't have a communal cemetery. I also learned that people almost never move from one house to another because their family members are buried on the property. Perhaps this is the reason Samoans don't or can't sell their houses. The traditional belief is that the deceased will protect the rest of the family. Who wants to buy a house with someone else's relatives buried in the front yard?

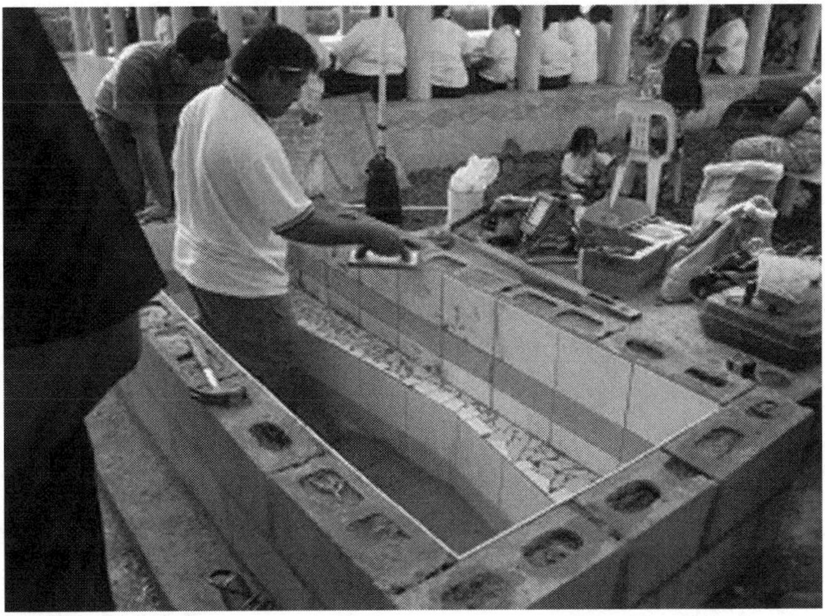

Building a tomb.

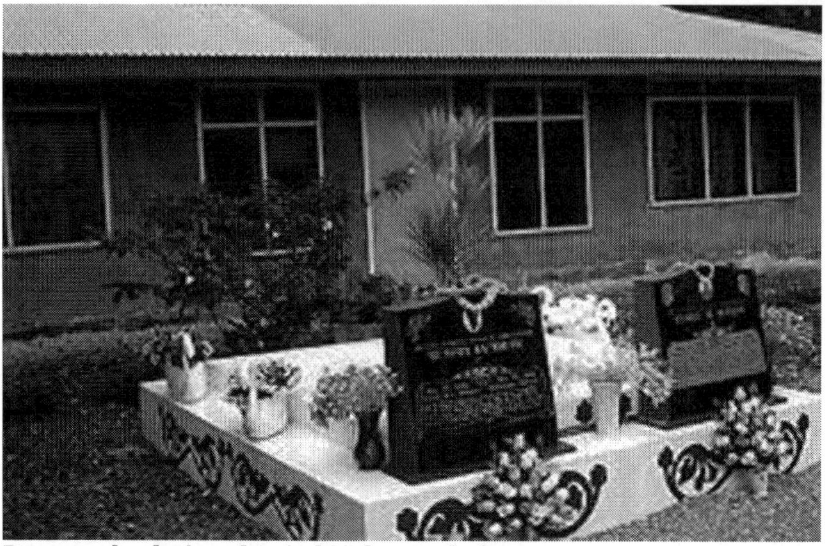

Deceased relatives buried in front of a house.

Throughout the funeral ceremony I attended, there were ladies who sat in the *fale* and sang songs, all from memory, with no accompaniment and in perfect harmony with one another. I was told that they'd been singing off and on during the night as well.

I mostly sat by myself, observing. At noon, I ran into a doctor from the hospital who told me that the departed was a distant cousin of his. He helped me with a plate of food. It was buffet style and included taro, *fa'i* (an unripened banana baked in an *umu*), *palusami* (a spinach-type dish made with coconut milk), pork, chicken, *sapasui* (chop suey noodles) and corned beef.

After lunch, amidst the singing, I bid goodbye to the doctor as I inconspicuously and quietly walked down the steps of the *fale* and onto the path lined with coconut trees that led out to the road and back to my hotel. It was truly a well spent day witnessing a very different funeral from ones I was familiar with.

Chapter 8

The Hong Kong Restaurant

AFTER TWO WEEKS OF HARD WORK, the chief of the hospital, Dr. Sua, invited all of us—including all the local doctors at the hospital plus most of the administrators—for dinner at the Hong Kong Chinese Restaurant, one of the most popular restaurants in Pago Pago. The Samoans loved their all-you-can eat lunches and dinners.

The Hong Kong Chinese Restaurant was situated not far from the museum in the center of Pago Pago. The exterior walls were painted green, and the doors and windows red. Above the entrance door was a four-foot carving of a dragon painted gold.

The owners, Mr. and Mrs. Lo, greeted us at the door with big smiles. Victor looked to be a man is his early or mid-fifties and his wife Tina was perhaps a few years younger.

As we entered the restaurant, I noticed that the inside was decorated with red lanterns, with one above each table. By the cashier was a tank of beautiful silver Arowana fish, a fish considered to be good luck because the color represents the metal silver, and in Cantonese it means *money*.

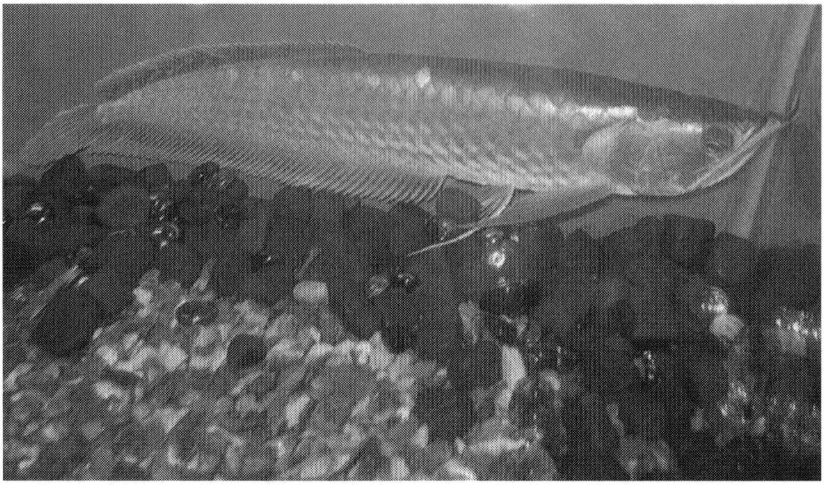

Silver Arowana fish at the Hong Kong Chinese Restaurant.

The U.S. representative for Samoa, a non-voting position in Washington, D.C., happened to be home and was at the restaurant that evening. Mr. Eni Faleomavaega welcomed us with a short speech and gave each of us one of his latest CDs—he was also a talented musician. After the speech, he sang a popular Samoan song as he strummed his guitar. All the Samoans at the restaurant sang along.

After we were all seated, hot and sour soup was served. This was made with shredded pork, mushrooms and eggs, and seasoned with cilantro and green onion. Usually tofu was also among the ingredients, but because it was Samoa, they couldn't easily get a hold of tofu.

The long buffet table was full of food of every description. The most popular dish was the deep fried salt-and-pepper pork chops. A close second was the deep fried whole chicken. The fried noodle and fried rice were also popular.

Victor Lo soon learned that I was from Hong Kong and came by to introduce himself. He was a slim man with dense black hair that stopped about an inch from his eyebrows. He spoke decent English and was interested in how I ended up in Pago Pago.

"Dr. John Paopao, the plastic surgeon who organized this visit, is from here," I answered. "We were suite mates in medical school and we became good friends. How did you end up running a restaurant in this part of the world?" I asked with a smile.

"Dr. Hung, as you know, we Hong Kong people fear the communists," he replied. "When we had the opportunity to immigrate, we took it. How Tina and I got here is a long story about fate.

"You know the ENT specialist at the hospital, Dr. Henry Lo? He helped us get here. He's my distant cousin. You see, his older brother Daniel Lo came here in the 1950s. How Daniel got here was never clear to me. I heard that their grandfather had been an indentured laborer here and when his contract was up, he returned to China with some money. I think Daniel was able to come here because of this connection.

"After arriving from Hong Kong with some money, Daniel opened the largest general store in Pago Pago. He became influential in this part of Samoa because he got to know the officials and often gave discount to their families.

"There was an American woman, a senior official here. In the 1950s, I think this part of Samoa was run by the Americans, specifically the U.S. Navy. From what I understand, this woman, Mrs. Campbell, a divorcee, was really influential in American Samoa. Somehow, she and Daniel met. Later they got married. Sadly, this American woman came down with ovarian cancer and was very sick for a long time. Daniel took good care of her for many years. Their love story was well known in American Samoa and the people here all thought very highly of Daniel.

"Daniel's brother Henry had graduated from the Sun Yat-sen University medical school and was stuck in Guangzhou, China working in a government hospital for a pittance as an ENT doctor. Life was miserable and there wasn't enough to eat. Using his influence, Daniel was able to get his brother to Pago Pago. The government even made an exception for him to practice medicine here, as his credentials weren't recognized in American Samoa.

"It was Daniel's connections that enabled my family and me to immigrate here, too.

"Our first choice was of course America," Victor added. "But without a great deal of money, we didn't qualify for any immigration scheme and so we came here. We learned that after a number of years, we would be permanent residents of American Samoa and we would be able to go to the U.S. I've known people who have done just that.

"It's confusing, because American Samoa is under the U.S., but somehow their immigration laws are different. It's much easier to come here. We hope in a few years, we can move to California. We have two children studying in California now. We know that for their sake, America will be a better place for them to settle down," he finished.

By now, I was almost finished with the soup. "This is delicious," I exclaimed.

Victor laughed. "Dr. Hung, as someone from Hong Kong, you know this isn't the best hot and sour soup you've ever had."

"It's really quite good," I protested.

"You're lucky because you are educated," he commented. "I never went to university so there aren't that many jobs I can do. This is just a way of making a living. So far, we manage. We have to be resourceful because the people here aren't that wealthy and they eat a lot. The profit margin is very slim. Luckily, the vegetables are very inexpensive here and the frozen meats from New Zealand and America aren't too expensive, so we can still make a profit."

"How did your children like school here?" I asked.

"Coming from Hong Kong, school was really easy for them here. Both of the kids graduated as valedictorian of their class. Our older son is now studying at the University of California at Los Angeles and our daughter just joined him a few months ago. We're lucky that our children will have all the opportunities Tina and I didn't have because our families were poor and our parents didn't take education seriously," sighed Victor.

"I'm very glad to hear that your children are doing so well," I said.

"Dr. Hung, if you have time, come visit us. We will steam a grouper for you. One of the luxuries of living here is that delicacies like fresh grouper cost a fraction of what it would in Hong Kong. Tina and I have steamed fish almost daily. They say that eating fish will lead to a long life," Victor chuckled.

One of the hospital administrators, Mr. Tuimavave, was also a talented musician and could do the fire dance. He showed us a video of a performance he'd done not long ago at a wedding.

Dr. Lo, the ENT specialist and Victor's distant cousin, soon joined us. He and Victor seemed like good friends. With not many Cantonese-speaking people in American Samoa, they appreciated each other's friendship.

As we conversed in Cantonese, which I hadn't done in many months, I felt at home with these people.

Victor was complaining about how much the local people could eat. "As you can see, all of them have their plates full," he remarked. "Each man, and many women too, can eat at least a pound of food. It's a good thing frozen pork and chicken from America cost so little compared to Hong Kong. On average, we get a pound of pork or chicken for less than two dollars. I don't even know how they make any money shipping the meat all the way here." He shrugged and added, "I understand that the quality of meat shipped here isn't the best. But as Chinese cooks, we have means to make such meat taste good."

"I thought the pork chops were delicious," I declared. "They were tender, juicy and full of flavor. The fried chicken too was mouthwatering, and the beef with broccoli was fantastic."

Victor smiled and said, "You know there's a secret to making cheap beef taste tender and juicy like it's the best cut. I learned from a chef in Hong Kong. Of course, you know that you have to cut the beef against the grain. And it needs to be tenderized. The most important process is massaging the meat, adding a little baking soda and then a little corn starch. Before you stir fry the meat, you should also add some sesame oil and massage it again. When you cook it, just stir fry it at high heat for a minute or so. In most cases, that will make even the toughest beef taste good."

"Don't the Samoans like seafood?" I asked. "I don't see much seafood on the table."

"The sad thing is that we can't afford to serve fresh seafood in a buffet like this, which we can only charge $9.99 for," sighed Victor. "Fresh seafood is expensive compared to the frozen meat and chicken. The fried fish you see on the table came from somewhere else, frozen also."

After a while, I joined John and the other fellows from Hawaii. John was asked to give a speech. He was full of humor and talked about his happy childhood and how happy he was to see many of his old friends again.

That was our goodbye dinner. The following day, we headed back to Hawaii.

Chapter 9
Trip to Apia

IN 2014, JOHN DECIDED TO ORGANIZE another medical mission, this time to Apia, the capital of Samoa (formerly Western Samoa). My other projects were going well, so I decided to join his group, which was composed of the same cast of characters who went to American Samoa a decade or so ago, with one more addition—Dr. Gosh, a urologist from Hilo.

On my flight to American Samoa over 10 years earlier, I was fortunate that even though I was in the economy class, I had an aisle seat in both directions. Some of the fellows weren't as fortunate and also had big people sitting next to them, which made the flight very uncomfortable. On this trip, I decided not to take any chances and paid twice as much to fly business class.

I usually like to get on a flight around mid-morning or noon so I'm well rested when I begin my journey, but in this case there were only three flights a week and they all left at 1 am. I had tried to sleep during the day without success. As we sat around waiting to board, we were told that the flight would be delayed at least an hour.

I was glad I'd decided to fly business class—I wasn't in any shape to sit in a small seat for the next six hours. Having learned his lesson from being cramped and surrounded by large people on previous trips with John, the urologist was also flying business class and was seated next to me. Dr. Gosh was from India and had come to the U.S. for his internship and residency. After his urology residency at the Mayo Clinic in Minnesota, he decided to open an office in Hilo, which had no urologist at the time. He was well read and knowledgeable about world affairs, and extremely interesting to talk to. We talked about the world, the U.S. and Asia, and agreed that in spite of the problems in the U.S., especially with gun violence, it was still the best place to live.

"I really can't think where else I could live, and I've travelled a great deal all over the world," I announced.

"James, I totally agree with you. I think America has been so wonderful to us," Dr. Gosh responded.

The flight attendant brought us another glass of champagne. "God bless America!" I exclaimed, raising my glass.

Dr. Gosh raised his glass and said, "Yes, God bless America and all the good people in this wonderful country."

We laughed and finished our drinks in one gulp.

After two glasses of champagne, I felt drowsy and soon fell into a deep sleep.

The flight was smooth and we arrived in Samoa on Sunday morning at 7 am. The main international airport, Faleolo International Airport, is a 40-minute drive west of the city. Samoa's major domestic airlines, Polynesian Airlines and Talofa Airways, service the airport. However, from Honolulu, we had to fly with Fiji Airlines, which made a stop at Apia on its way to Fiji.

John had arranged for a van to take us to our accommodations. I had hoped to stay at the legendary Aggie Grey's Hotel, but unfortunately it was closed for major repairs after being severely damaged by floods and a category 5 cyclone.

The ride to the hotel was very scenic. We passed several villages along the way, and I noticed that each house had at least one *ulu* (bread fruit) tree, a mango tree and several coconut trees growing in the front yard. In contrast to the coconut trees in Hawaii, those in Samoa were much lower, and the fruits were smaller and more yellow on the outside. Someone explained to me that because Samoa is often hit by cyclones, through evolution the coconut trees became lower, as only the shorter trees survived over the course of millions of years.

The main thing that struck me on the drive was the sheer number of churches visible in the villages. I went on to learn that there were approximately 3–4 churches per village in the 300 or so villages across Samoa, and that around 98% of the country's population was devout Christian.

On arrival in Apia, we checked into the Annabelle Inn, a house that had been converted to an inn, located on a frontage road facing the extensive beach.

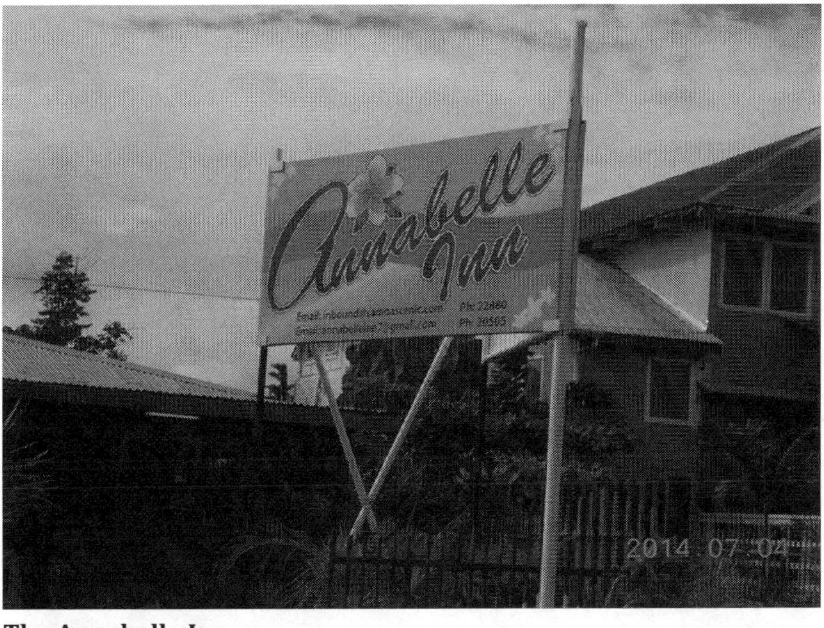

The Annabelle Inn.

We sat down in the lobby and each of us had a cold green coconut water. The ceiling fans were working hard to keep us cool.

I had exchanged some money at the airport and was inspecting the local currency. "Do you guys know how the Samoan money got its name?" I asked.
Everyone seemed puzzled and no one could come up with the answer.

"Think! Look at the bill—that'll give you the answer," I laughed.

Still no one could figure it out. They all laughed when I explained, "It's their way of saying 'dollar'. There's no 'D' in the Samoan alphabet, so they used 'T', and hence, 'Tala'."

A U.S. dollar was to equivalent to about 2.5 Talas at the time.

My heart sank as I checked into my room. It was tiny, no larger than ten feet by ten feet, and it had a rusted ceiling fan. The inn wasn't air-conditioned. Unlike Hawaii, Samoa was a great deal more humid and the cooling trade winds weren't as regular as in Hawaii.

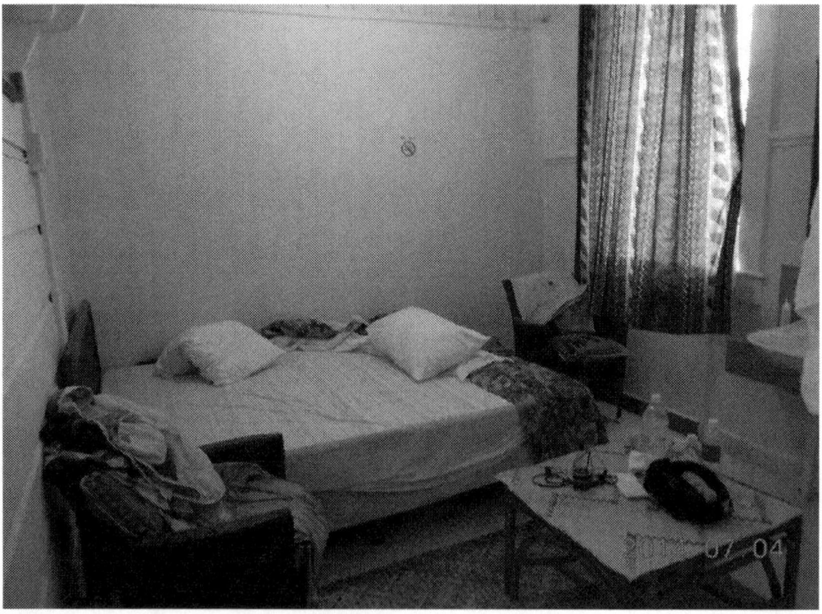

My room at the Annabelle Inn.

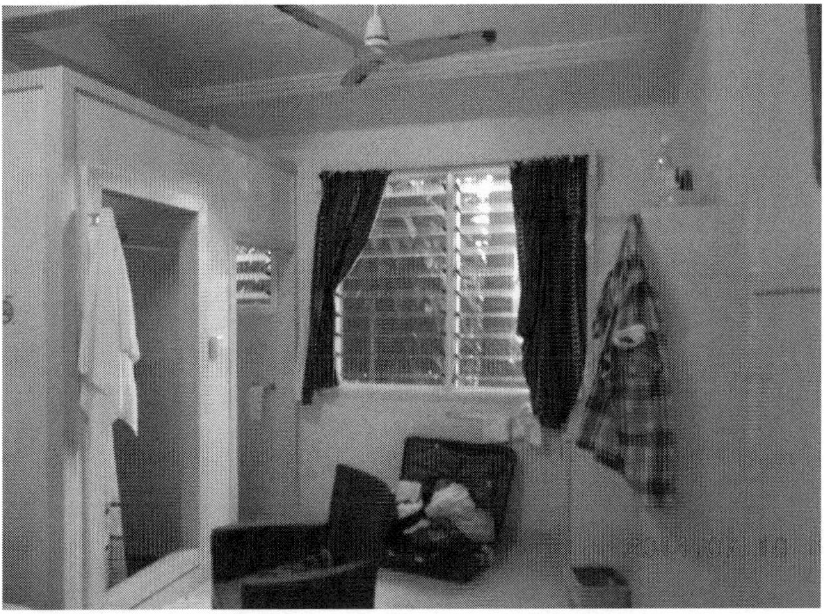

My spartan accommodation with a rusty ceiling fan.

In my travels, especially on medical missions, I always tried to stay in a comfortable place because I wanted a good night's sleep before work the following day.

My first impression of the room at the Annabelle wasn't good. My first night was a nightmare, as the feral dogs outside the inn barked almost constantly all night. *(Samoa has problem with feral dogs. Many families use dogs to guard their homes, as crime in the country has been on the rise.)*

To add to the annoyance, it was mango season, and throughout the night the mango trees over the inn would drop a fruit now and then, hitting the corrugated tin roof with a loud bang. It was not a restful night.

After the second night, I got more used to it. By the third, I was liking the place and couldn't understand why I was upset when I first arrived.

The five Samoan women on staff were wonderful. I learned that they were the staff from the now-closed Aggie Grey's Hotel.

***

Apia is located on the central north coast of Upolu, Samoa's second largest island, situated on a natural harbor at the mouth of the Vaisigano River. The harbor was the site of a notorious naval stand-off in March 1889 in which seven ships—from Germany, the U.S. and Britain—refused to leave the harbor, even though a typhoon was clearly approaching, lest the first one to flee lose face. All the ships sank or were damaged beyond repair, except for the British cruiser *Calliope*, which managed to leave port traveling at a rate of one mile per hour and ride out the storm. Nearly 200 American and German lives were lost.

Apia was originally a small village, from which the country's capital took its name. The modern city of Apia was founded in the 1850s, and has been the official capital of Samoa since 1959. Apia Village still exists within the larger city, which has grown into a sprawling urban area that encompasses many villages, with a population of just under 40,000 inhabitants.

The city's historical haphazard growth from village to colonial trading post to the major financial and business center of the country has resulted in major infrastructure problems. Issues with flooding are commonplace during the wet season, given that the city is built in a low valley. The increase in vehicle ownership has resulted in traffic congestion in the city streets and the need for major projects in road-widening and traffic management.

Some of the Apia's early wooden colonial buildings are still standing, most notably the old courthouse from the German colonial era, with a museum on the upper floor.

The city's Catholic cathedral, the Immaculate Conception of Mary Cathedral, was dedicated on December 31st, 1867. It was pulled down mid-2011, reportedly due to structural damage from the earthquake of September 2009. A new cathedral was built and dedicated on May 31st, 2014, just two months before we arrived.

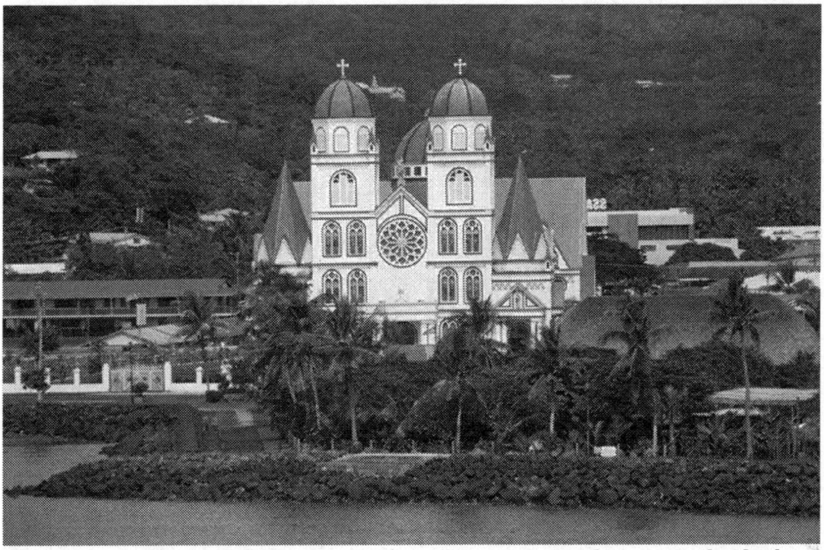

The new cathedral: The Immaculate Conception of Mary Cathedral.

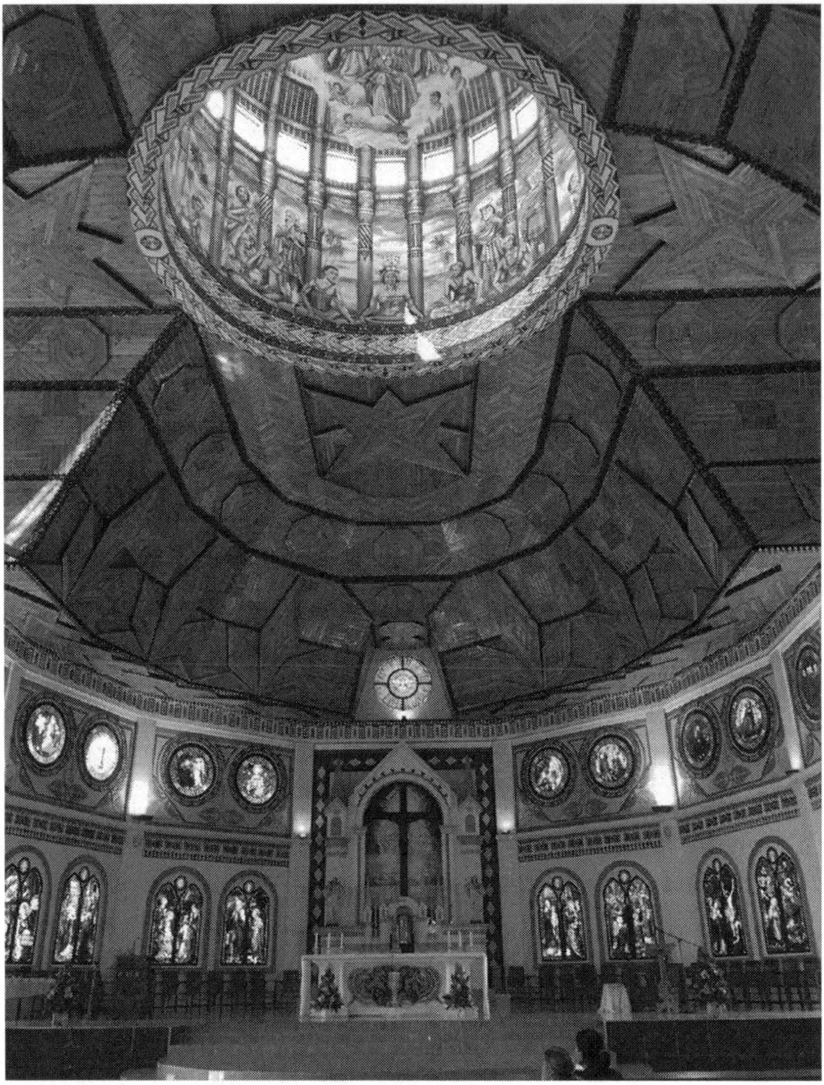

The beautiful interior of the Cathedral.

Thirty percent of the businesses in downtown Apia are owned by one East Asian family. Ten percent of them are owned by Europeans, while the other 60% are owned by the local community.

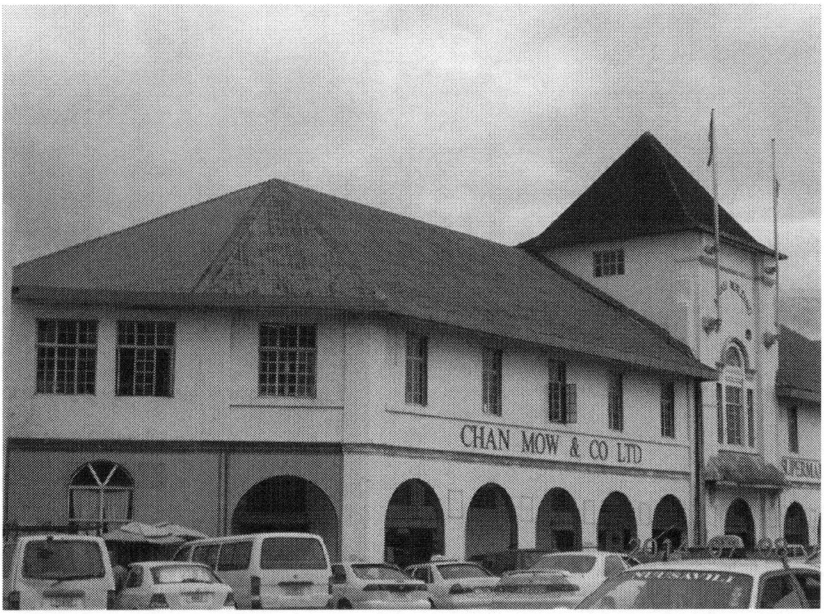

The Chinese Family that owns 30% of the downtown business in Apia.

Apia harbor is by far the largest and busiest harbor in Samoa. International ships carrying containers, LPG gas and other fuels all dock there. Ferries to Tokelau and American Samoa also depart from the harbor.

The country has no trains or trams, but is served by an extensive, privatized bus and taxi system. People commonly walk around the town, and even some distances outside it. There are few bicycles or motorcycles, with mostly cars and trucks adding to traffic congestion in the city streets. I found it very easy to get around in Apia, especially on the brightly painted buses that cost very little.

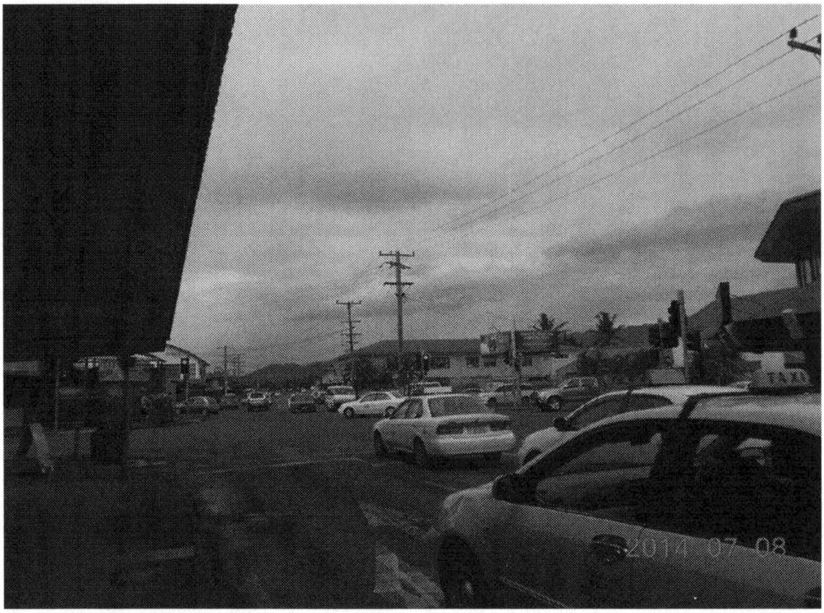

Downtown Apia on a rainy day.

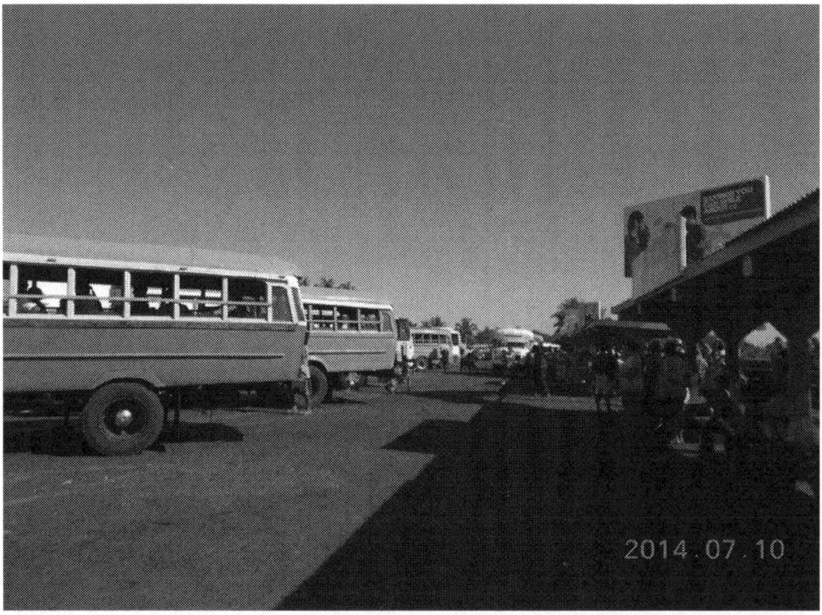

The Bus Terminus, with buses converted from trucks and vans.

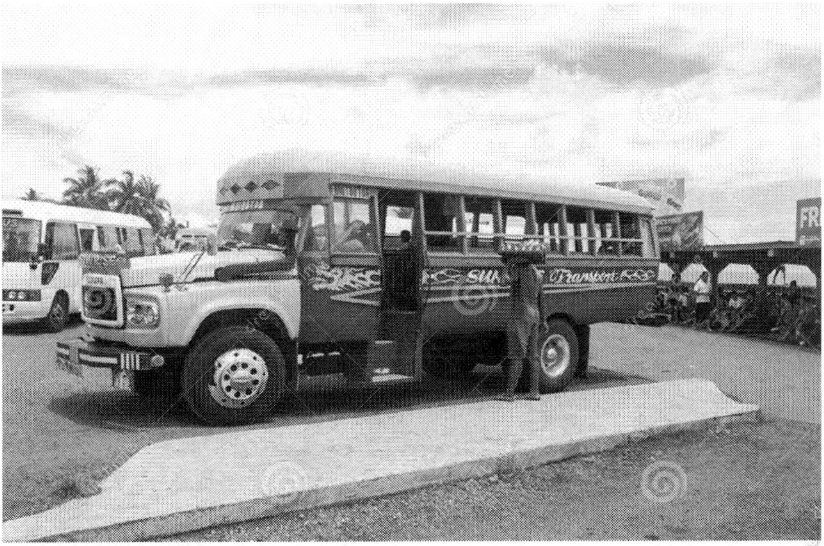

A typical local bus.

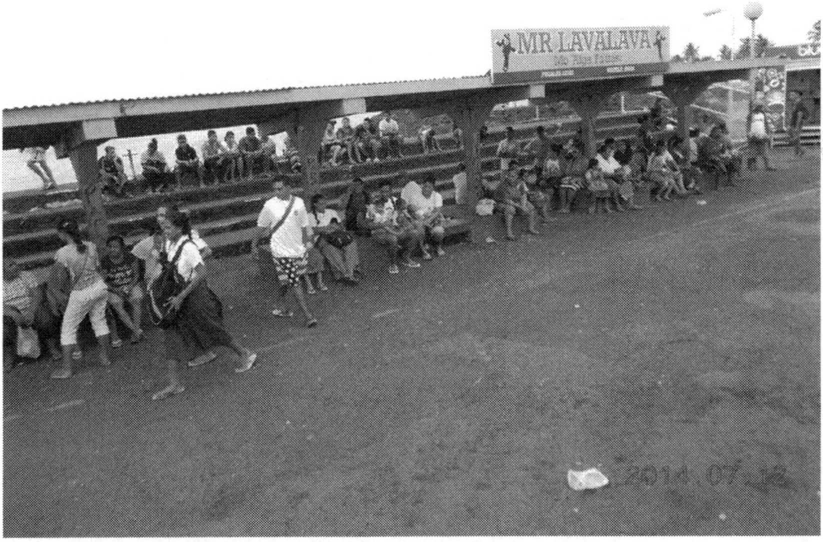

The bus terminal next to the fish market.

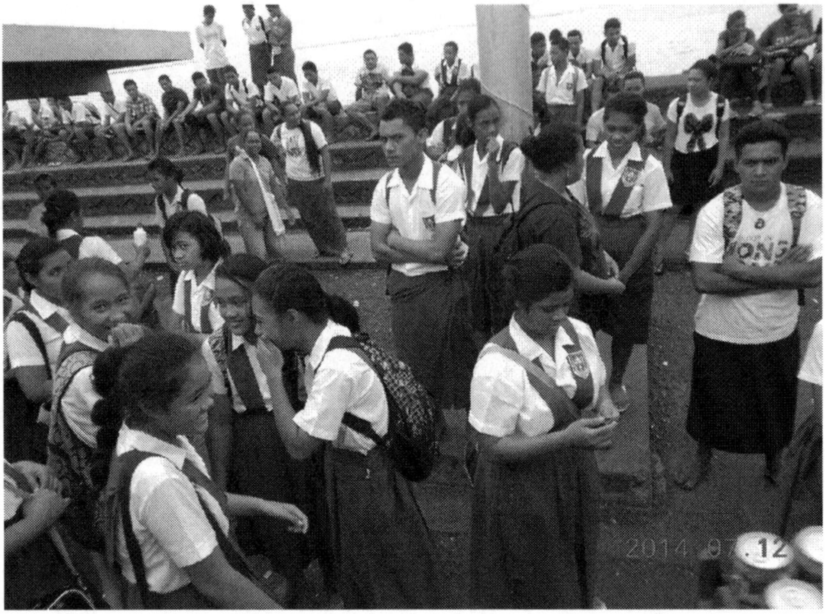

Students waiting for the bus.

Students wanting to continue their education after high school have options to stay in Samoa. In addition to the National University of Samoa, there is also the University of the South Pacific School of Agriculture, both located in Apia.

A major primary and secondary school in the city is the private Robert Louis Stevenson School. It's known as Samoa's upper class school, due to many children of Samoa's wealthy classes attending it. It was named after Scottish-born writer Robert Louis Stevenson, who spent the last four years of his life in Apia, and is buried on Mt. Vaea overlooking both the city and the home he built, Vailima, now a museum in his honor.

***

One day, after a hard day's work, we all sat in the lobby of the inn and had a Vailima beer. A Samoan man wearing a short-sleeved white shirt and a blue *lava lava* sat down with us and began talking to Dr. Gosh as if he was an old friend. The rest of us soon joined in the conversation. Half an hour later, this man open his bag and displayed a number of *lava lava*. He explained that because we were such good folks, here in Samoa doing good deeds, he was selling them at cost. Not wishing to embarrass Dr. Gosh, most of us bought one. After paying him, the man packed up his goods and left.

"How long have you known that man?" I asked Dr. Gosh.

Dr. Gosh looked bewildered and replied, "I've never seen this man before. I thought he was one of you guys' friends."

We all burst out laughing.

Dr. Gosh added that a couple hours earlier, while taking a walk on the beach road, a Samoan man had approached him saying he was the immigration officer when he arrived. In order to avoid any problems leaving the country, this man advised Dr. Gosh to pay him five Talas. He complied, not knowing that he was a con man.

"It's amazing that these sorts of scams are so common in Samoa now," John lamented.

I was surprised. I'd always thought of Samoans as such honest and kind people. I kept imagining it to be how Hawaii was a century ago. For the most part, the people were exceedingly generous, friendly and honest. As in any country, there are always a few bad apples that try to take advantage of others.

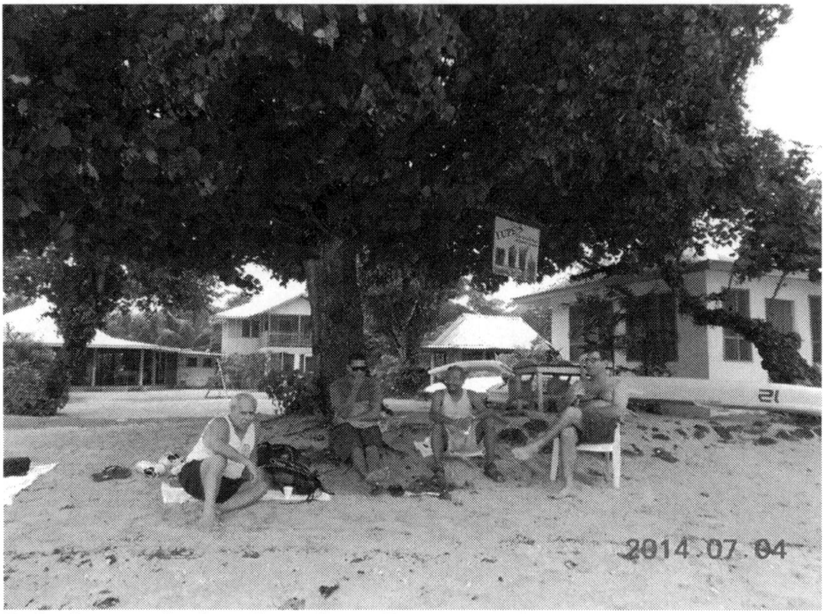

Relaxing on the beach under a Banyan tree.
From left: Dr. Paopao, a local doctor, Dr. Gosh and Dr. Garin.

Chapter 10

The Tupua Tamasese Meaole Hospital

ON TUESDAY MORNING, our team was the center of attention. The Tupa Tamasese Meaole Hospital at Motootua was hosting a continuing education conference at 8 am in the lecture hall. The hospital's auditorium was brand new and impressive, enough to hold about two hundred people.

Most of the staff, doctors, nurses, administrators, and other allied health personnel filled almost the entire auditorium. The head of the hospital gave a short introduction of our team and I was to lead off the conference by giving a lecture on the latest treatment of diabetic retinopathy. The incidence of diabetes in Samoa was the same as in American Samoa—almost half of the population—so the number of patients with diabetic retinopathy was very high.

I explained that the treatment was one of the success stories of eye care, with an almost 100% success rate. I emphasized that in 2014, no one should go blind because of diabetic retinopathy. Unfortunately, some still did in Samoa because the patients lived in isolated villages, and by the time they saw a doctor they had already lost their vision. The damage done to the retina by diabetes was non-reversible. It was of utmost importance that the treatment be performed before patients began losing their vision.

I then showed a short video of how a laser treatment was done. It took from 15 minutes to half an hour and didn't involve any cutting. Generally, no anesthesia other than a few drops of anesthetic on the eye was required. As I wrapped up the presentation, there were several questions from the audience. Many of them had no idea how the treatment was done before this and were truly surprised by how easy it seemed.

Dr. Douglas Johnson, the dermatologist from Honolulu, then gave a review of common skin diseases.

After the conference, we headed for different clinics where we were needed.

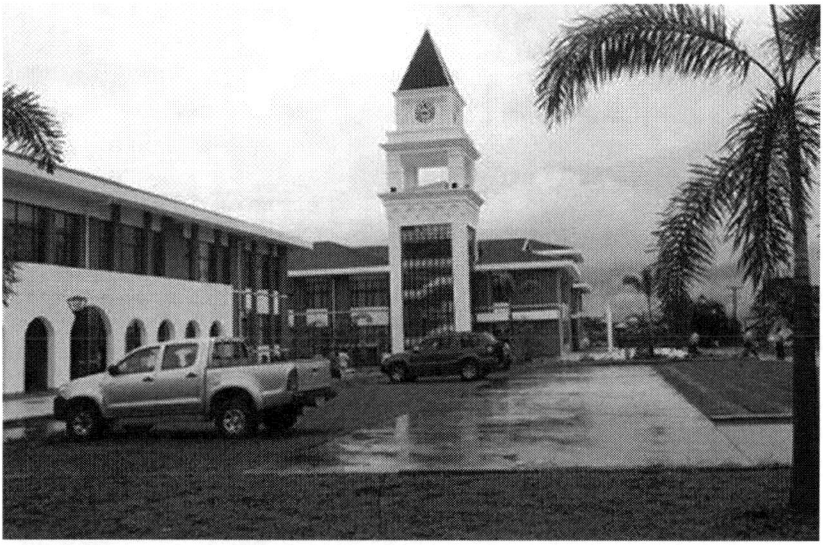

The brand-new Tupua Tamasese Meaole Hospital.

The Tupua Tamasese Meaole Hospital at Motootua looked impressive from the outside, although parts of it hadn't yet been completed. Chinese construction workers could be found in different areas of the building. The hospital was being built by the Chinese government as a goodwill gesture, with a 30-year loan set up for financing

I'd recently read that the Chinese government had been very generous to Samoa. Some critics thought this was setting Samoa up to owe debts it couldn't repay. In addition to the hospital project, the Chinese were helping construct a new port costing a few hundred million U.S. dollars. Many felt that a population of 200,000 didn't need such an expensive port, and there was no way the country could repay the loan.

I heard stories about how the Chinese bribed government officials with extravagant trips to China—the same officials who would be deciding on the contracts for different projects.

The Tupua Tamasese Meaole Hospital is connected to the other Samoan hospitals and clinics. The specialists working in the hospital extend services to the Malietoa Tanumafili II Hospital at Tuasivi on Savaii (the smaller Samoan island) and the district hospitals.

The hospital is also the headquarters of the Samoan Ministry of Health, and is a teaching hospital for the medical school next door. Medical students from other countries can take rotations in the different departments.

I was very interested to visit the medical school. The Oceania University of Medicine (OUM) is a Samoan-chartered medical school operated through a public-private partnership between the Government of Samoa and e-Medical Education, LLC, a Florida-based company. It was founded in 2002 by philanthropist Taffy Gould, a handful of Australian doctors and others to fill a void: a shortage of medical personnel in the South Pacific.

The OUM curriculum is divided into two phases: preclinical and clinical. The preclinical phase is offered via distance learning and lasts a total of 96 weeks, followed by 72 weeks of hands-on clinical rotations at the hospital, and at some regional teaching hospitals.

The National Health Service is the main health care provider for the residents of Samoa, operating all hospitals and health centers. The main hospital, the Tupua Tamasese Meaole

Hospital, provides most of the care, and also houses one of Samoa's several pharmacies.

In addition to the main hospitals, there are also several health clinics and general practitioners located around Samoa. In many rural areas healthcare facilities are very basic.

Tertiary care is mainly provided through arrangement with the New Zealand health care system.

The eye clinic was closed Friday afternoon, so I decided to spend some time in the Emergency department. I'd always kept up with general medicine and was comfortable treating the common conditions often seen in the E.R.

A fisherman arrived with a cut on his right cheek after another fisherman's hook caught it and got stuck. The cut was about an inch long but not deep. After anesthetizing the patient's cheek with Lidocaine, I placed four stiches to close it. There was only one physician working in the E.R. that day and it was busy. I was glad to pitch in and enjoyed playing a 'real doctor' instead of just an eye doctor!

I learned from one of the nurses that many patients showing up at the E.R. had severe complications of their diseases, such as presenting themselves in florid septic shock due to festering diabetic wounds that had been treated at home with topical traditional remedies for weeks, sometimes even months.

I was surprised that many of the patients knew only very basic phrases in English and certainly not enough to answer specific questions about their health. I was also shocked by how seriously unwell many of them were upon arrival at the E.R.

At about 3 pm, a very ill 49-year-old woman was brought in by her family with generalized abdominal pain and distension, as well as severe fatigue and altered mental status. The E.R. doc had seen this patient before and the diagnosis was very late stage polycystic kidney disease, where the kidneys almost filled the entire abdominal space.

The strong influence of Samoan family culture was apparent in this case. The patient had only sporadically been in contact with the healthcare system, and several months previously her family had refused dialysis, so she was now in acute renal failure. In discussing her case with the doctors, the family explained that the patient was the youngest sibling in her family, thus her older siblings had the final say in decisions relating to her care.

The E.R. doc called in the only surgeon at the hospital to evaluate if this woman needed surgery. Dr. Poniponi was a tall, solid, athletic man of about 50 with gray hair down to his shoulders. I learned that he handled almost all the surgical cases, including amputations in diabetic patients, complicated gynecological operations, urological emergencies and, in one instance, major open bowel surgery for a five-week-old neonate.

I was surprised to hear that in spite of the large number of patients on dialysis, there was no nephrologist in the country, and the patients were managed by a general internist and a couple dialysis technicians.

I also learned that there was no pathologist in Samoa. The previous one had left over a year ago and they hadn't yet found a replacement. The problem was that the government had little success in keeping many of the doctors. I was told that the hospital was top heavy, with many high-paid administrators, while the doctors earned not much more than school teachers. It seemed that many of the administrators got their positions through political connections and had little respect for the doctors, treating them as their subordinates.

The woman with the polycystic kidney was admitted and the family agreed to let her be dialyzed and perhaps to have the mass removed.

At about 4 pm, a slim man who looked to be in his late sixties or early seventies was dropped off by his family. I was called to check on him because his right eye was closed from large growth involving the both the upper and lower lid, extending to his right ear and most of the right side of his head. Some areas were ulcerated and bleeding. It was obviously some sort of tumor. I'd never seen one that size.

Dr. Doug Johnson was still seeing patients in the dermatology clinic, so I decided to consult him. Usually he and the pathologist from Honolulu, Dr. Tom Namiki, worked together.

Dr. Namiki had developed a method to determine what sort of tumor we were dealing with, and he could give Doug the results in an hour or two. With no pathologist in the country, we were lucky to have Dr. Namiki as part of our team. An orderly took the patient to the dermatology clinic for a biopsy.

Later that evening, at dinner, I learned from Dr. Namiki that the man had basal cell carcinoma (also called basal cell skin cancer), the most common type of skin cancer. About 8 out of 10 skin cancers are basal cell carcinomas.

These cancers usually develop on sun-exposed areas, especially the face, head and neck. They tend to grow slowly. If left untreated, basal cell cancer can grow into nearby areas and invade the bone or other tissues beneath the skin. Sadly, for this man, the tumor had spread to the muscles, his right earlobe and upper and lower eyelids. He needed extensive surgery to remove all the cancer. If not removed completely, basal cell carcinoma can recur.

After John examined him, a plan was set to do the surgery sometime the following week. As the tumor had spread to a large area, John suspected he would need some skin graft from the patient's forearm or thigh. In the meantime, the hospital would do further workups on him such as X-ray and MRI to determine if the tumor had metastasized to other parts of the body, like the bone or liver.

I felt bad that this poor man had sought medical help so late in the disease. As with many Samoans living on the other island,

Savaii, coming to Apia was a major ordeal. They had to take a ferry, then find their way to the hospital. Many of them lived in remote villages and had little means; making such a trip would be something they couldn't afford.

I learned that the Samoan health system was about to get an injection of doctors from China to help alleviate the shortage in medical personnel. An agreement had been signed between the Chinese government and the Samoa Ministry of Health.

The *Samoa Observer* reported that the Chinese Medical Team (C.M.T.) Agreement would see Chinese doctors brought in to work where needed. The Minister of Health, Dr Talalelei Tuitama, said it was a significant contribution provided by the Chinese government to complement the efforts by Samoa to address the shortage of medical doctors in a number of specialized areas.

The paper said China's ambassador to Samoa, Wang Xuefeng, announced that there would be four medical teams with six medical personnel in each team sent from Jilin Province in Northern China over a two-year period. The ambassador also said that since the 1980s about 100 medical professionals had traveled from China to work in various Samoan hospitals.

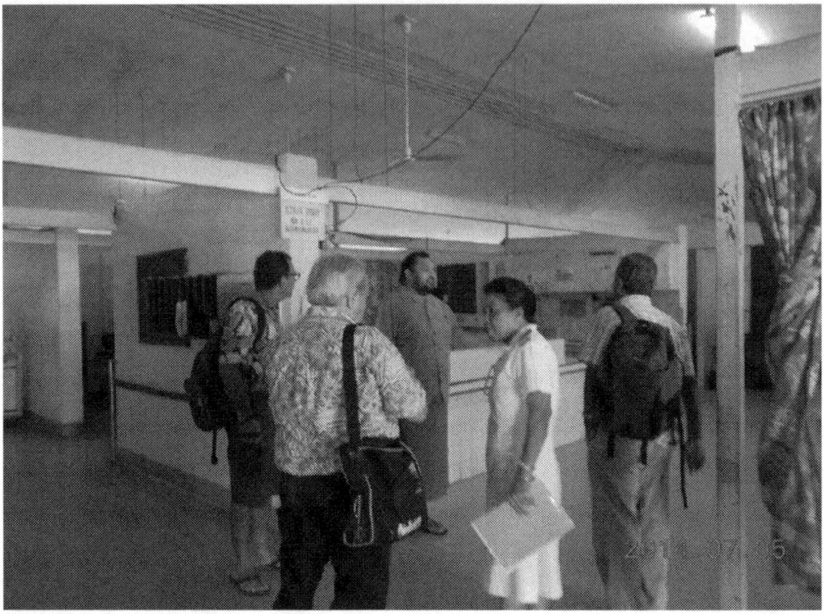

Making rounds at the hospital.
John (Dr. Paopao) talking to the head nurse, in the foreground with his back to the camera.

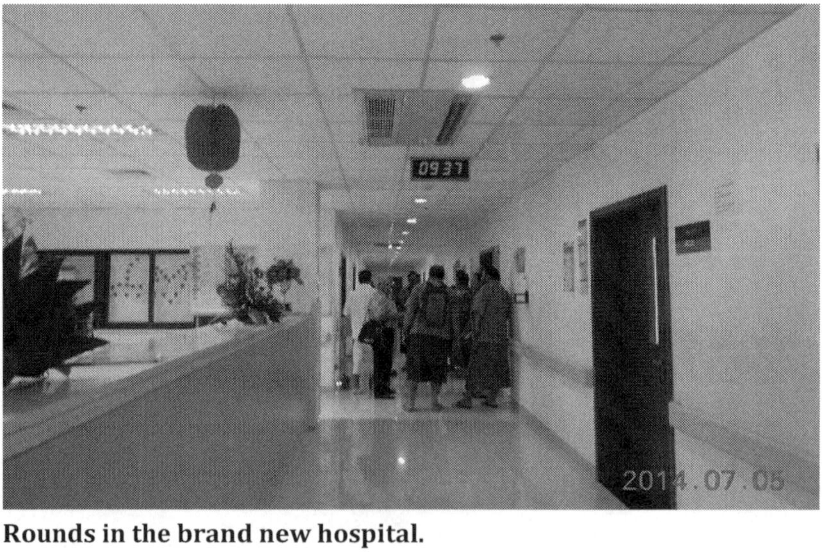

Rounds in the brand new hospital.

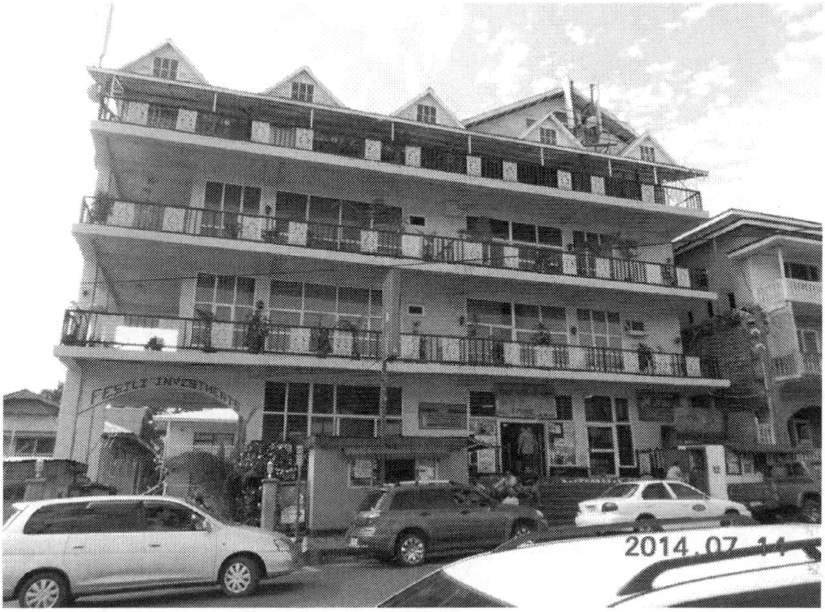

Apartments and businesses across from the hospital.

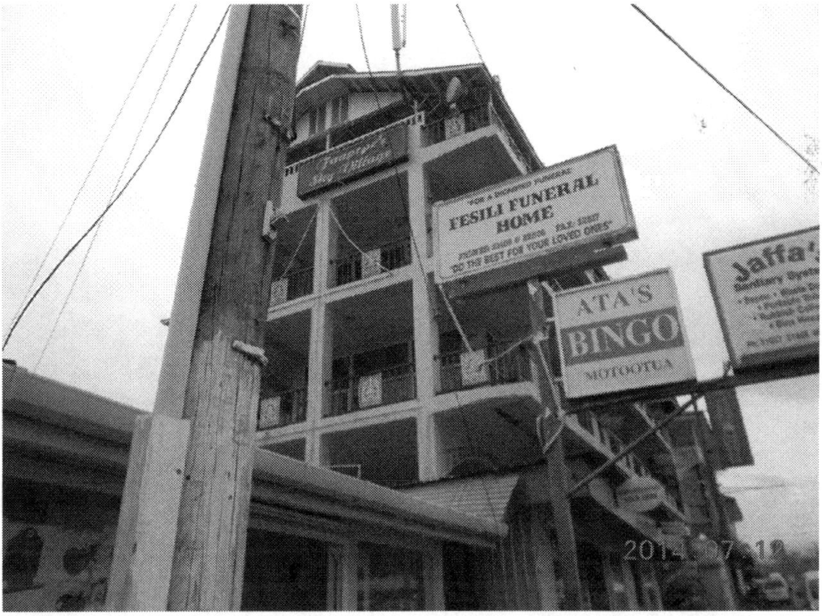

Funeral home and other businesses across from the hospital.

We worked hard for two weeks. On Friday evening, we were invited to a feast. On Saturday, we were invited to a dinner show at a hotel, which included the famous Samoan Fire Knife Dance. The dance was spectacular. One of the dancers was a boy of 10 or 11 years old who was the champion of his age category for that year's Fire Knife Dance competition. The Samoan culture was a macho one, and the Fire Knife Dance was a good example of that.

In spite of having grown up in American Samoa, I noticed that John was also well known to the people of Samoa. To most Samoans, the division is artificial, and the two countries are one people and one culture.

Chapter 11
The Eye Clinic

MONDAY MORNING, I WAS ANXIOUS to get started at the eye clinic. After two eggs, some bacon and hash browns washed down with black coffee, I took a taxi to the hospital, with my large suitcase containing a laser machine in tow. The taxi driver didn't know where the eye clinic was, so he dropped me off in front of the main hospital. It turned out that the eye clinic was still in an old wing of the old hospital about half a block away.

Pulling my suitcase, and after asking several people, I found my way to the entrance of the clinic. It was 8:30 am, and everything was still closed. Waiting at the door was an elderly Caucasian man, of no more than five feet tall. In Samoa, where most people were over six feet tall, he really was conspicuous. With a big smile on his face, he extended his right hand to shake mine.

"Good morning," he greeted. "You must be one of the doctors from Hawaii."

He was a compact man wearing a light blue short-sleeved shirt and a pair of long khaki shorts. His sparse hair was mostly white and he wore a pair of gold wire-rimmed glasses.

"Good morning. Yes, I am one of the doctors," I replied with a smile. "My name is James Hung."

"My name is Peter Bonadelli," he said. "I'm here as a patient. I'm being treated for glaucoma. I'm usually the first one here because there's no appointment system—it's first come, first served. So I usually get here around 8:30 to beat the crowd."

"Are you visiting Samoa or do you live here?" I asked.

"I've been in Samoa for six years now," he responded. "How I ended here is a long story."

I glanced at the locked clinic doors and smiled. "I have time." We both sat down on the steps as I listened to Peter's tale of how he ended up in Samoa.

"I taught at Sophia University in Tokyo for many decades," he began. "My wife taught there too. After we retired, we returned to Boston where we grew up. But I found my life purposeless. I felt like a useless old man. We had three teenage grandkids, but they were so spoiled and they really didn't need me. Their parents bought them all sorts of gifts, and they had no idea what real life was like.

"I was only 74 and I felt really restless. My wife and I visited Hawaii and thought maybe we could find some part-time work there. I interviewed at the Hawaii Pacific University, but they had no opening for someone like me who specialized in Japanese culture. My wife and I also found Hawaii too commercialized and too noisy. We checked out Samoa, and I fell in love with the place and decided to make this my home. After a few months, my wife couldn't stand it here, so she returned to Boston," remarked Peter.

"How did you end up as a specialist in Japanese culture?" I asked.

"Dr. James, it's another long story. When I was a young man, I was fascinated by the Japanese people, their language and their culture. So, when I finished high school, I learned that Boston College had just begun a program in Japanese studies. I was one of their first students. It was 1955, not long after World War II. After I graduated from Boston College, I went to Tokyo and enrolled in their Ph.D. program. After my Ph.D., I stayed at Sophia University and taught for over 30 years. My then girlfriend, who had graduated with a degree in English language from Tuft's University, joined me in Tokyo where she taught English at the same university.

"Our two children grew up in Japan, but they went back to Boston for college and they stayed there. I guess they didn't care for Japan as much as I did," he chuckled.

By now it was 9 am, and the doors of the clinic opened. While Peter and I talked, a line had been forming and there were already over 20 people waiting.

The head nurse, a young Samoan woman, greeted Peter, who introduced me to her.

"Yes, we're expecting you, Dr. Hung," Sophie said with a smile.

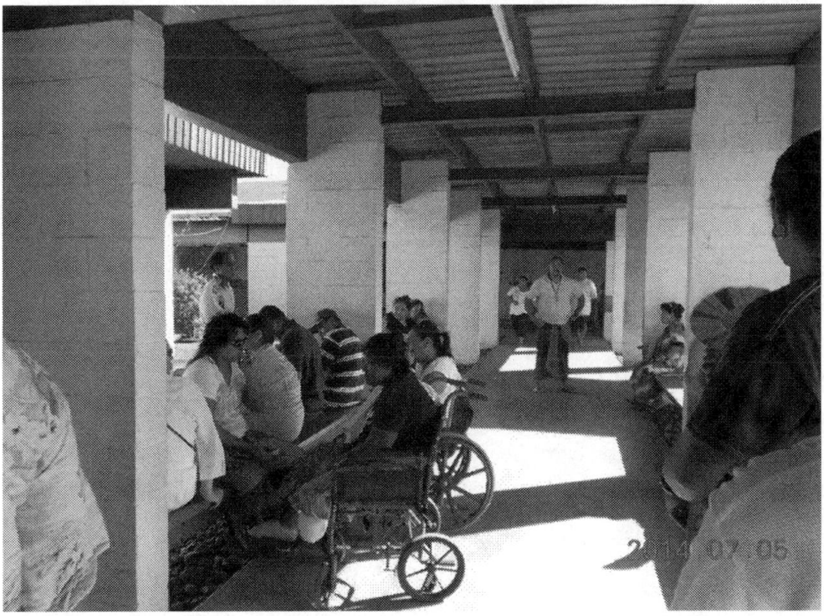

Patients waiting in front of eye clinic.

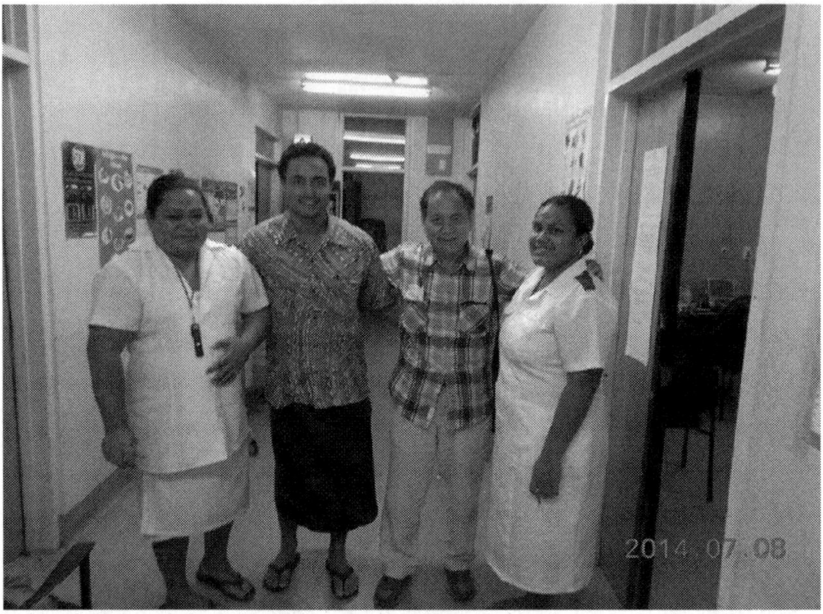

From left to right: Head Nurse Sophie, Dr. Robert Schultz, the author and another nurse.

Peter was ushered into the first examination room. Sophie checked his eye pressure, which was 15, an acceptable number.

"Dr. Hung, we have a number of patients waiting to see you for treatment of diabetic retinopathy. They've all been screened," Sophie explained.

Dr. Taloa, the only ophthalmologist in the country, arrived at the clinic and came to meet me. She wore a very friendly smile. Standing next to her, Peter and I felt like midgets. She was almost six feet tall.

"Dr. Hung," she said, "I have a house officer here who would like to shadow you. He's interested in going into ophthalmology. I hope you don't mind if he hangs around you."

"Of course not," I replied. "I'd love to show him how to use the laser."

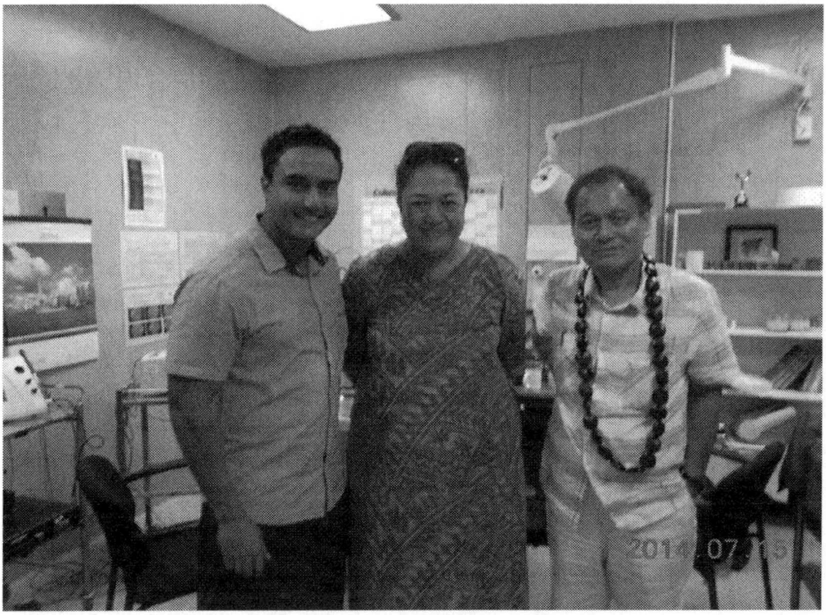

From left: Dr. Robert Schultz, Dr. Taloa and the author.

The young house officer, Dr. Robert Schultz, was part German and had graduated from Otago University medical school in New Zealand just a few months earlier. Samoa had paid for his education, and now he had to repay the country by working there for at least two years.

Dr. Taloa examined Peter and assured him that he was responding to the medications and doing well. Before he bid me goodbye, he invited me to dinner the following day.

My clinic day went very well. Setting up my portable laser, which I'd done many times in different countries, was no problem. In addition to being the surgeon, I was also the technician. Even as a young boy, I'd been fascinated with how machines worked and had taken a few clocks apart. Unfortunately, I couldn't put some of them back together!

Before buying the laser, I had asked the technician many questions, and essentially got a crash course on how to troubleshoot if the laser didn't work. Since then I was always able to repair any minor problems, and fortunately I hadn't had any major ones.

I did laser treatments on 10 patients that morning. Robert helped me explain to the patients what I was doing, and he himself was very curious and inquisitive about the process.

Dr. Toloa was busy with the other clinic patients, while I helped with the backlog of patients needing laser treatment for diabetic retinopathy.

At noon, Sophie brought Robert and me fried chicken for lunch. Dr. Toloa had a hospital meeting and couldn't join us. The chicken was quite tasty, and we washed it down with ice cold Cokes.

Robert was a very personable young man, handsome and strong. He had inherited the best features of his Samoan and German heritages.

"How do you like working here?" I asked him.

"It's not easy," he admitted. "After being in New Zealand for years, I'm used to a more organized society. The major problem in this hospital is the management. I don't think they have the most qualified people running the hospital. Many of them got their jobs because of who they know. It's frustrating."

"I'm sorry to hear that," I responded.

"They have trouble keeping good doctors here," Robert lamented. "The pay is so much lower than in New Zealand. Even an intern there makes three times as much as a qualified full-time physician here.

"It's demoralizing to study hard for so many years, and then return to Samoa with a doctor's qualification, but only have the salary of a school teacher.

"After my two years here, I'm definitely not sticking around," he added. "I know I'm not patriotic in that regard, but I have to take care of myself and my family first. It's not just the money. I've talked to many staff physicians here and they all seem unhappy because there are so many politics involved in running the hospital. It's all about who you know.

"I'm applying for a position in New Zealand and I hope to get into a training program in ophthalmology. It's one of the most competitive specialties to get into," Robert remarked.

"How did you end up in medical school at Otago?" I asked.

"Each year, the Samoan government takes the students with the best marks in the eleventh- grade exam—equivalent to the O Level in the U.K.—and puts them into a special school. There they have the best teachers to prepare them for the equivalent of an A Level exam. Those who score the highest are sent to New Zealand on full scholarships. I was lucky that I had one of the highest scores in my class and I got my first choice to study medicine at Otago," he explained.

"What was it like at Otago University? I understand that it's the best university in the country," I remarked.

"It was extremely competitive," he replied, nodding. "We were in the so-called First Year Health Science curriculum. There were almost 2,000 of us. We took the same courses, seven very difficult courses, and at the end of the year we would apply to the second year of medical school, dental school, or pharmacy and other health-related fields. They took less than 300 for med school, and only 50 for dental school. Almost half of the students in first year were hoping to get into medicine. Naturally, many of them were disappointed. Talk about a pyramid system of the worst kind!

"It was stressful," he continued. "The workload was so heavy that there was no time for anything else. The bad thing was that we knew we were competing with each other. It was a zero-sum game. If someone else did better than you, then your chance of getting into medical school lessened. I was lucky to do well enough to be selected for the medical school."

At 1 pm the afternoon clinic began. I turned on the laser machine, and again calibrated the settings and resumed treating patients. The afternoon went quickly, and we treated the last patient just after 5 pm. Robert insisted on giving me a ride back to my hotel.

The following day, a Tuesday, was the morning conference at which I gave the lecture on the latest information on diabetes and diabetic retinopathy and its treatments. After the conference, I returned to the eye clinic, which went much like the previous day. The treatments on all the patients went smoothly. Again, Robert insisted on taking me back to the inn.

Peter had invited me to dinner at an oceanfront restaurant not far from the Annabelle Inn. It was a nice walk along the beach. Peter and another man were sitting down, each sipping a Vailima beer, when I arrived at the restaurant. Peter stood up and greeted me, shaking my hand.

"Dr. James, I would like you to meet another Peter, Peter O'Sullivan, the U.S. Consul General in Samoa," Peter introduced.

"Nice to meet you, Your Excellency," I said with a smile.

Both Peters laughed. "Just call me Big Pete," chuckled Mr. O'Sullivan. "As you can see, I'm much taller and bigger than Peter. Since there aren't that many Americans here, the expats call me Big Pete, and Peter, Lil Pete."

We all laughed. Big Pete was well over six feet tall, and weighed at least 200 lbs.

I learned that as Samoa was a small country, the person representing the U.S. was not an ambassador, but rather only a Consul General.

"Do they call the Consul General 'Your Excellency' also?" I asked.

"Here, people just call me Pete or Mr. O'Sullivan," he answered.

"I'm so glad Big Pete got transferred here last year," Peter exclaimed. "We see each other a couple times a week, and we talk about everything under the sun."

"Yes, I'm so glad to have Pete here," the Consul General agreed. "When I first met him, he was like my long-lost friend. I was so glad to leave Zimbabwe where I'd been for four years. I was the deputy ambassador there—or the deputy chief of mission, which was my real title.

"Life was so hard there," he added. "I really missed the ocean—as you probably know, Zimbabwe is a landlocked country. I've never seen so much misery in one place, and it's all because of bad people running the country."

"Would you happen to know a woman by the name of Rebecca Zeigler who also worked at the embassy in Harare?" I asked. "She's the daughter of a very good friend of mine."

"Oh yes, I know Rebecca really well," he replied. "She's in charge of the scholarship department. Every year she selects a number of the brightest high school graduates to attend university in the U.S, free of charge. She's been in Zimbabwe for years. She really helped me out when I first arrived there."

"What a small world it is!" I exclaimed. "Of all the places in the world, you and I know the same person in Zimbabwe."

The waiter came to take our dinner order, and we all ordered the seared tuna. When the food arrived, I was surprised to see a large chunk of beautiful tuna done to perfection. I ordered a green coconut water to go with the meal. As we were finishing our dinner, some of the other members of our team, Drs. Gosh, Namiki and Johnson showed up and joined us.

As we sipped our beer, the sun was just setting. The orange glow slowly sank into the horizon. Surrounded by coconut trees and the soothing sound of the waves, and conversing with very interesting people, I had such a memorable evening. We sat and talked until the restaurant closed at 10.

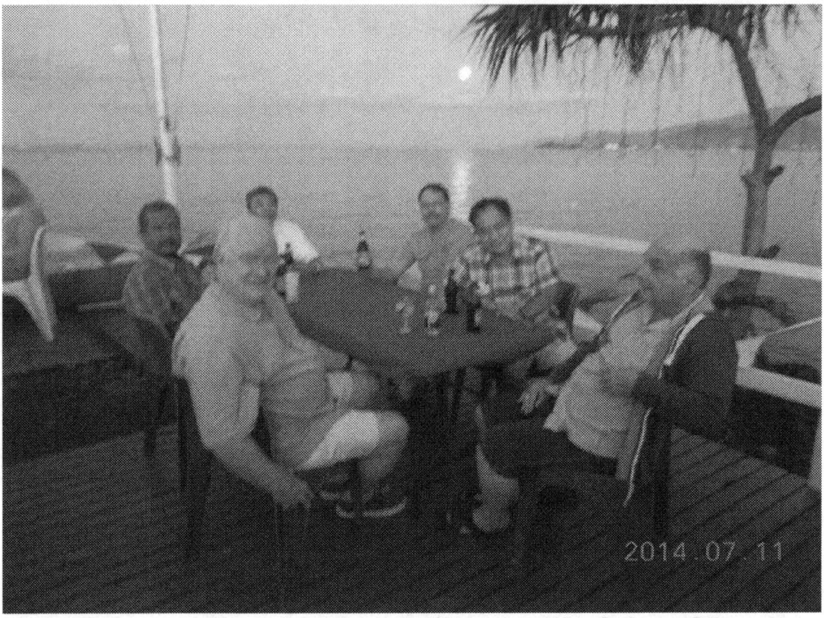

The U.S. Consul General, Peter O'Sullivan, on the left, and Peter Bonadelli on the right. In the background from left: Drs. Gosh, Namiki, Johnson and the author.

Chapter 12
The Paintball Injury

BEFORE I RETIRED FROM PRIVATE PRACTICE, I was getting tired of the rat race. There was too much paperwork—so much that it was taking away from time I could be spending with my patients.

The working environment for doctors was getting worse each year. I was fortunate to be in ophthalmology and didn't feel as harassed as the primary care doctors. Some of my friends who graduated from medical school in the mid-1970s were working over 60 hours a week, almost as hard as when they were interns, just to make ends meet: to pay their rent, nurses and other office expenses on the highly reduced reimbursements they got from HMOs, Medicare and Medicaid. And then a huge part of what was left went to pay for malpractice insurance.

Some of their frustration was more than just the money. It was the intrusion on their autonomy. Many of them spent endless days and long years acquiring an extraordinarily specialized skill, only to find themselves being told by some young administrator, often with little medical training, how many minutes they could spend with a patient, how long they could keep a patient in the hospital and what sort of treatment they were allowed to give.

With the EHR (Electronic Health Records) being made mandatory by the government, many doctors spent countless hours keying information into the computer that few would ever read. A case in point was when I saw my internist, who didn't get up from her chair at the desk even once, and only asked questions as she keyed in my responses. She never examined me and there was little eye contact, as she was busy looking at the computer screen. The human touch of being a medical doctor was gone.

I was luckier than most because I truly did enjoy my practice and I quit before the EHR became mandatory. I decided that it was time for me to do something else, such as writing and doing more charity work in developing countries.

Going on a medical mission is different because you know you're doing something good, helping people who would otherwise not get the help, making a difference in people's lives.

The two weeks I spent in Apia were educational for me as well. I was glad that, with my experience, I felt I could handle any eye problem. Many general ophthalmologists weren't comfortable treating the retina. Since I'd taken a fellowship in retina surgery, I was comfortable dealing with almost any eye condition, except perhaps the repair of a tear duct in an eyelid injury or a fracture of the eye orbit.

In the past, if I had a patient with a lacerated eyelid involving the tear duct, I would invariably refer him or her to someone with more experience, like a doctor who'd done a fellowship in ocular plastic surgery. If I had to, I could get the job done. But if there was someone with more experience available, it wouldn't be fair to the patient to handle it myself. It would take me longer, and probably wouldn't be as good a job.

Similarly, if I had a patient with an orbital fracture, I would certainly refer him or her to a maxillofacial or ocular plastic surgeon, because I had minimal experience in repairing them.

After one day at the eye clinic, I took one of the colorfully painted city buses, which cost me about 50 cents, back to the Annabelle Inn. The five of us were having dinner at the inn's small dining room that evening. As usual, I ordered tuna fish, seared. Because tuna was abundant and inexpensive, and caught in the morning, I was certain that Apia was one of the best places in the world to enjoy fresh tuna.

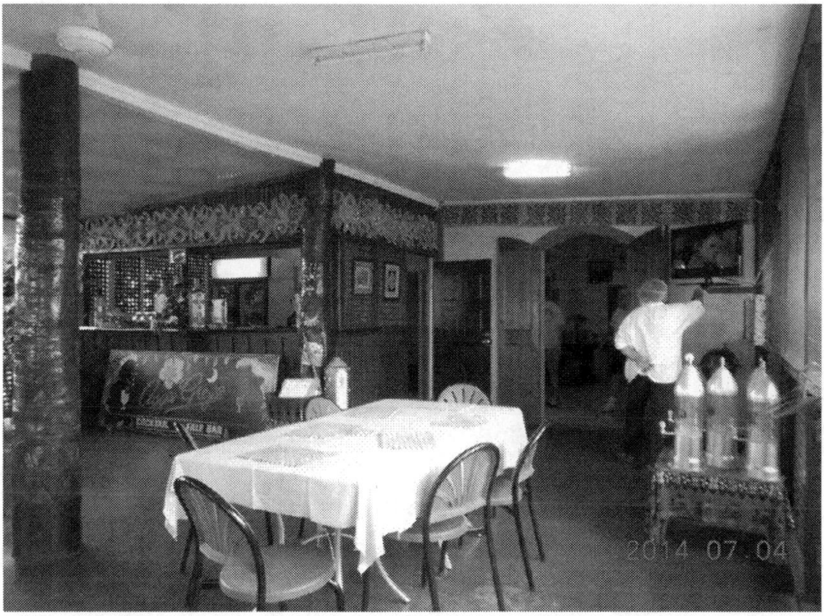

Dining Room at the Annabelle Inn.

At the table, John was telling us about the two-year-old girl whose cleft lip and palate he'd repaired that day. Doug Johnson was relating all the unusual skin diseases he and Dr. Namiki had seen in the dermatology clinic. He also surprised us by saying that he'd gone to the leprosy clinic for consultation. I had no idea there were still patients with leprosy, as I thought the disease had been eradicated.

Nowadays, the medical community in the U.S. generally avoids using the word leprosy and the official name is Hansen's disease. But in Samoa, the clinic for such patients was still called the leprosy clinic.

It turned out that my friend Peter Bonadelli was in charge of the leprosy clinic, even though he wasn't a physician or nurse. The clinic was sponsored by a Catholic NGO, and Peter was very involved with several NGOs in the country. The patients were usually treated by a doctor from the Philippines, where the disease was still endemic. This doctor would see the patients every few months. In between, Peter was overseeing the patients' welfare, helping them with financial aid and advice. He had requested that Doug come see some patients with skin problems.

As we enjoyed our seared tuna and garlic mashed potatoes, washing the food down with ice cold Vailima beer, the front desk receptionist, a slim young Samoan woman named Milly, came by the table and said someone at the hospital wanted to speak to me.

I excused myself and went to the phone. It was Dr. Schultz.

"Dr. Hung, I hate to bother you," Dr. Shultz said apologetically, "but I have a patient I don't know what to do with. Dr. Taloa is helping her husband [a Lutheran minister] at his church and suggested that I call you to see if you'd be interested in taking care of him."

"What sort of problem does the patient have?" I asked.

"It's a 15-year-old boy. He was hit in his right eye with a paintball. I can't see the pupil. I think there's blood inside the eye," Dr. Schultz answered. At that point, Dr. Schultz only had a couple of months' experience working in the eye clinic with Dr. Taloa, and knew very little about ophthalmology.

I told Dr. Schultz that I'd be happy to help with the patient, and that I'd be at the eye clinic in about half an hour.

I returned to the dining room to finish my dinner, and explained to the gang that I had to leave and take care of an eye patient.

By the time I arrived at the eye clinic in a taxi, it was after 7 pm, and already dark. Dr. Schultz was waiting for me at the door, while Sophie was in the examining room with the patient.

The boy was sitting in a chair with his parents next to him. He looked more mature than 15, over 6 feet tall and at least 200 lbs. He had a blue plastic eye shield covering the injured right eye. I learned that his name was Fred. He looked scared and had tears in his left eye.

Sophie introduced me to his parents. "This is Dr. Hung, an eye specialist from Hawaii. He's here for two weeks to help us. He is the best."

The parents stood up and shook my hand. They seemed educated, and later I learned that the father was a bank manager and the mother a school teacher.

"What happened?" I asked.

The father looked embarrassed and said, "It's all my fault. Last year when I went to Honolulu on a business trip, I bought four paintball guns, one for each of my two boys and their cousins. I told them they had to wear goggles when they played their war game. Fred took off his goggles to load paintballs when his cousin accidentally shot him. It looks like it hit the eye and now he can't see."

A paintball gun or paintball marker, is an air gun used in the shooting sport of paintball. Paintball guns use compressed gas, such as carbon dioxide (CO_2) or compressed air, to propel dye-filled gel capsules called paintballs through the barrel to hit a target.

The term "marker" is derived from its original use as a tool for forestry personnel to mark trees and ranchers to mark wandering cattle. When the gel capsule (paintball) hits the target, it bursts and the paint splatters.

"Let's see what sort of damage you have," I said to Fred, leading him to a chair in front of the slit lamp. I carefully removed the eye shield. The lids were a little swollen but not shut. With a sterile cotton tip applicator, I lifted Fred's upper eyelid to get a better view of his eye. I couldn't see the pupil and the eye seemed to be filled with blood, just as Dr. Schultz had said. I gently touched the eyeball and it felt soft, which meant there was a leak, i.e., a wound that was leaking fluid from the eye.

I moved Fred's chair closer to the table and placed his chin in the cup of the slit lamp. Even with the brightest light from the lamp, I still couldn't see the pupil.

I asked Sophie if there was an ultrasound machine for eyes in the clinic, which would help to assess the extent of damage, such as the amount of blood or if the retina was detached.

"Sorry, Dr. Hung," Sophie replied, shaking her head. "The machine broke a few months ago. We haven't been able to send it to New Zealand for repairs yet."

"The light's very bright," complained Fred.

"That's a good sign," I remarked. "It means your retina is probably alright."

I told Fred's parents that I'd treated similar eye injuries before. "I'm quite sure there's a wound at the limbus of the eye," I explained. "The limbus is the area between the cornea, which is the clear part of the eye, and the white of the eye. It's dangerous to try and examine it more because we may do more damage. What Fred needs is to be put to sleep for me to carefully examine the extent of the damage and repair it."

"When should it be done?" his father asked.

"As soon as we can—probably tonight," I replied. "We need an anesthesiologist. Sophie will do some calling around to see if one is available."

Sophie headed out of the examination room to make the calls, and I carefully put the eye shield back over Fred's eye. He was quiet and seemed frightened.

When Sophie returned, she announced that Dr. Wang, a doctor with the Chinese medical team, would be available to assist us.

Surgery was set for 10 pm. We couldn't do it earlier because Fred had eaten a hamburger around 3 pm, just before the paintball fight. If we tried to put him under anesthesia with food in his stomach, he might vomit and do severe damage to his lungs.

Dr. Wang arrived at the clinic in good time. She was a petite woman of about 40 years old. Her English was limited, but I was able to communicate with her in Mandarin and found out that she was from the Shanghai area. She inserted a needle into a vein in Fred's left wrist and began a normal saline drip, which was necessary so medication could be given to Fred intravenously.

Shortly after, a surgical nurse named Elizabeth arrived and began setting things up. When Fred was settled on the operating table, the surgical nurse handed Dr. Wang the vial of antibiotics I'd ordered, for her to infuse into Fred's IV. This was to prevent infection.

Next, Dr. Wang efficiently put Fred to sleep.

Dr. Schultz was in attendance and excited that he was able to participate in an eye surgery. I carefully cleaned the area around Fred's eyelid with betadine solution. Under the operating microscope, I was able to see a wound that ran from the 1 o'clock to the 3 o'clock area of his eye. The area in front of the pupil was filled with blood. With a blunt-tipped irrigating needle and syringe, I gently irrigated BSS (balanced salt solution) into the eye.

BSS is used to maintain the natural condition of the eye during surgical procedures.

Once the blood clot was removed, I was able to see the pupil, which was round, indicating that the iris wasn't damaged. To my relief, the lens behind the pupil was clear and unharmed. If the lens had been damaged, the surgery would have been more complicated. I'd have had to remove the damaged lens, and then decide if I should replace it with an intraocular lens during surgery, or wait until later, after the wound had healed.

I placed four very fine black silk sutures to close the wound and injected more BSS to re-inflate the eyeball.

With the indirect ophthalmoscope, I was able to examine the retina carefully and was very pleased to see that there appeared to be no further damage. If I'd seen blood in the vitreous, I wouldn't be able to examine the retina to tell if it was damaged. In the U.S., if there was blood inside the eye, we would use a vitrectomy machine to remove it. But there was no such machine in Apia. Luckily for Fred, his retina looked healthy.

The surgery took a little more than an hour.

I explained to Fred's parents that he was very lucky the damage wasn't more severe. Now, we just had to wait to see how it healed and make sure there was no infection.

A few years earlier I'd treated a boy who was also shot in the eye with a paintball gun. The paintball hit the center of this poor fellow's left eye and caused it to rupture. The damage was extensive. His lens was dislocated into the vitreous and I had to fish it out. He needed many more surgeries after that. The retina was also damaged. Initially I thought he would lose the eye, but eventually we were able to save it, although with only 20/200 vision, which is legally blind.

An accident like this involved several unforeseeable situations. In Fred's case, he just happened to have his goggles off when the paintball hit him. Usually the socket protects the eye, but the eye was hit instead. He was very lucky that the paintball probably hit at an angle, and not directly. If so, the damage would have been more severe, and more similar to the other boy's injuries.

By the time we finished, it was past midnight. Fred was admitted to the hospital to continue with intravenous antibiotics to prevent infection. His mother stayed with him while his father gave me a ride back to the Annabelle Inn. He was most grateful that we were able to save Fred's eye. If such an injury went untreated, as happens in some parts of the world, the eye would become infected and would eventually be lost.

I thanked Fred's father for the ride and crawled into my bed, quickly falling sound asleep, oblivious to the barking feral dogs and the falling mangoes hitting the corrugated tin roof.

Chapter 13
Dr. Paopao, the Plastic Surgeon

IN MEDICAL SCHOOL, one of the specialties that interested me was plastic surgery. I talked to Dr. Robert Flowers, the preeminent plastic surgeon in Honolulu at the time. He was philosophical about his specialty, gave me some advice, and left me with the impression that in order to be a good plastic surgeon, one not only had to be a good technician but also an artist who understood beauty as well. Feeling that I lacked the second quality, I chose orthopedic surgery, and later switched to ophthalmology.

For decades beginning in the 1950s, Dr. Ivo Pitanguy, a pioneering Brazilian plastic surgeon in Rio de Janeiro, performed face lifts, tummy tucks and other procedures on the rich, famous and royal from around the world. There were other surgeons just as good as he was technically, but he understood beauty, which made him the most famous and celebrated plastic surgeon in the world.

John impressed me as an exceptional plastic surgeon because he also understood beauty. He was an excellent oil painter of tropical flowers as well as a sculptor. I had observed him in surgery and was impressed with his calmness during the procedures and the purposefulness of each step. He always planned ahead before each case, making drawings of what he was going to do.

I was especially impressed by his repair of cleft lip and palate. It was like performing a miracle, changing a person's face from disfigurement to beauty. I think cleft lip and palate surgery are some of the most life-changing procedures one can do. The surgery changes the patient from having to hide his or her face to one full of confidence. We use the expression *to face the world* because it's our face we present to it. For those with a disfigured face, like a cleft lip and/or palate, facing the world wouldn't be easy.

In the U.S., nowadays, we rarely see someone with a cleft lip or palate. This is because all babies with the condition would have surgery long before they were one year old.

Sadly, in developing countries we still see children and adults with the disfigurement. For the unlucky ones who never have it corrected, life can be challenging. The condition not only leaves the person with a face that attracts negative attention, it also causes many other health issues.

I really felt bad for Fetu when I first saw him. The literal translation of Fetu is *star* in Samoan, but Fetu was no star. In fact, he had spent his life trying to hide his face.

The sad part was that the condition could have been corrected with surgery in one to two hours, which would have spared him all the humiliation, emotional suffering and health problems. Because of his disfigurement, Fetu never got married and worked as a laborer on the docks, helping the fishermen carry their catch to the market.

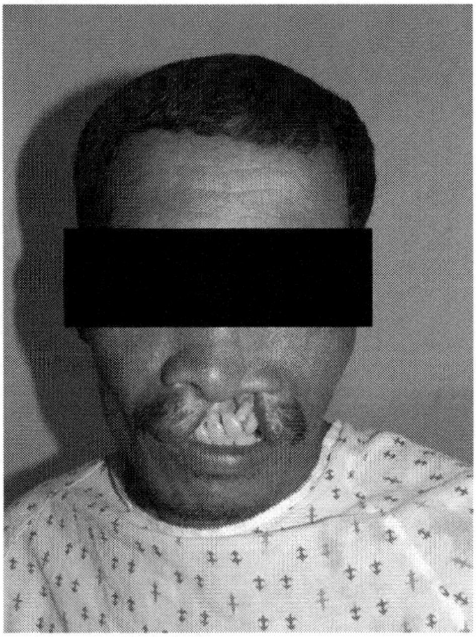

Dr. Paopao's patient, Fetu.

Fetu's cleft involved the gums, with several teeth tilted and out of position.

***

A cleft lip or palate happens when the structures that form the upper lip or palate fail to join together when a baby is developing in the womb.

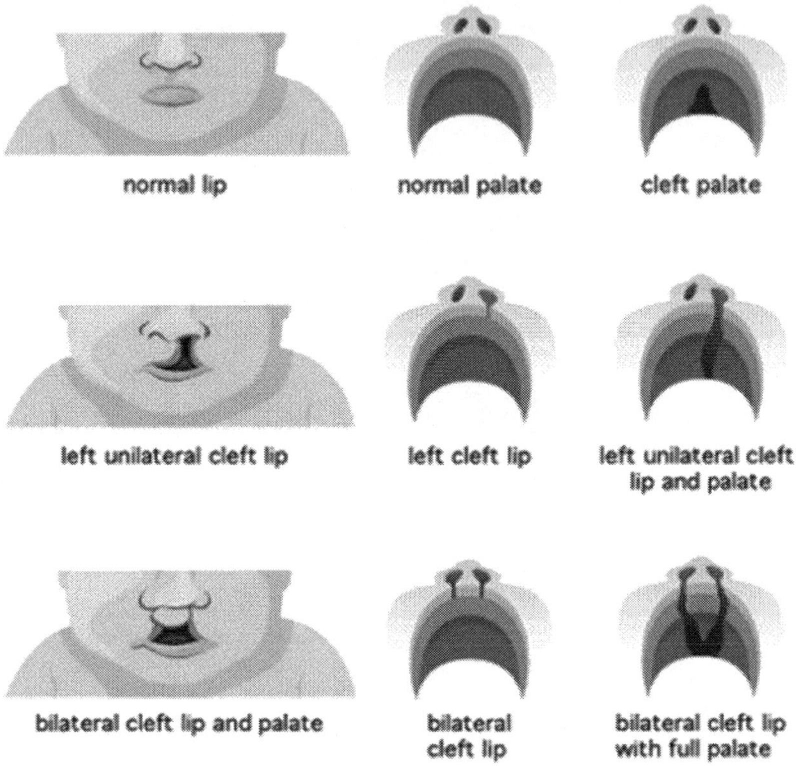

Types of cleft lip and palate.

The exact reason why this happens to some babies is often unclear. In a few cases, cleft lip and palate are associated with:

1. The genes a child inherits from their parents;
2. Smoking or drinking alcohol during pregnancy;
3. Obesity during pregnancy;
4. Lack of folic acid early in pregnancy, which is known to cause neural tube defects such as spina bifida. One study showed a strong association between maternal folic acid intake and the risk of a baby developing cleft lip and palate; or
5. Taking certain medicines in early pregnancy, such as some anti-seizure medications and steroid tablets.

In some cases, a cleft lip or palate can occur as part of a condition that causes a wider range of birth defects, such as 22q11 deletion syndrome (sometimes called DiGeorge or Velocardiofacial Syndrome) and Pierre Robin Sequence or Syndrome.

In the U.S., a cleft lip is usually picked up during the mid-pregnancy anomaly scan done between 18 and 21 weeks of pregnancy, although not all cleft lips will be obvious at this time. In cases where the cleft lip or palate doesn't show up on the scan, it's usually diagnosed immediately after birth or during the newborn physical examination done within 72 hours of birth.

An untreated cleft lip and palate can cause a number of issues, particularly in the first few months after birth, before surgery is done. They can include:

1. Difficulty feeding—a baby with a cleft lip and palate may be unable to breastfeed or feed from a normal bottle because they can't form a good seal with their mouth;
2. Hearing problems—some babies with a cleft palate are more vulnerable to ear infections and a build-up of fluid in their ears (glue ear), which may affect their hearing;
3. Dental problems—a cleft lip and palate can mean a child's teeth don't develop correctly and they may be at a higher risk of tooth decay; and
4. Speech problems—if a cleft palate isn't repaired, it can lead to speech problems such as unclear or nasal-sounding speech when a child is older.

Most of these problems will improve after surgery and with treatments such as speech and language therapy.

The majority of children treated for cleft lip or palate grow up to have completely normal lives.

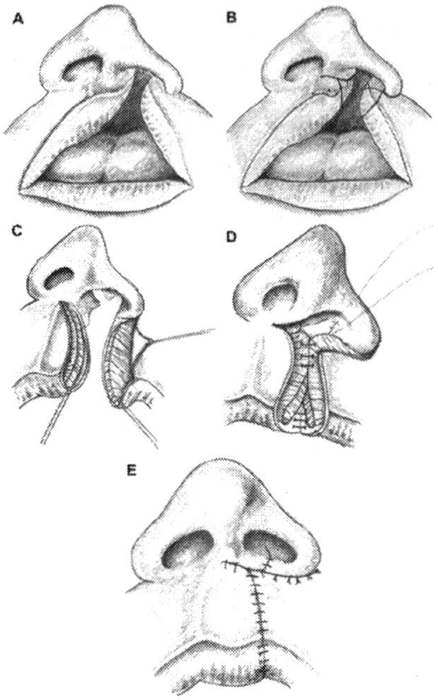

Surgery for cleft lip.

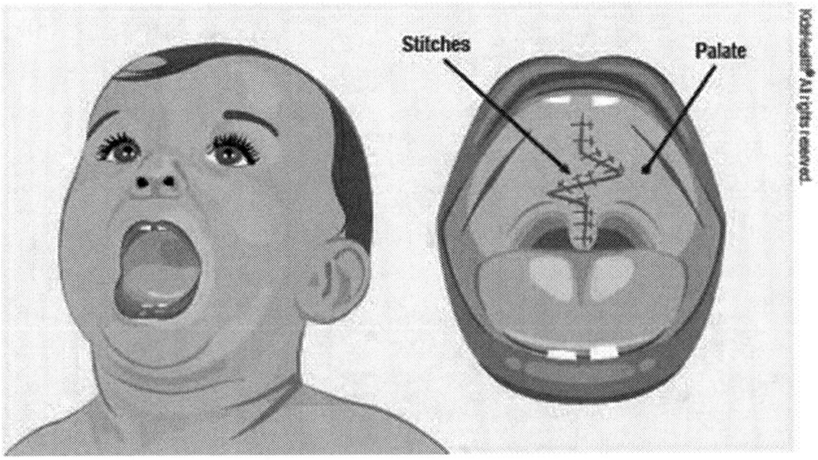

Surgery for cleft palate.

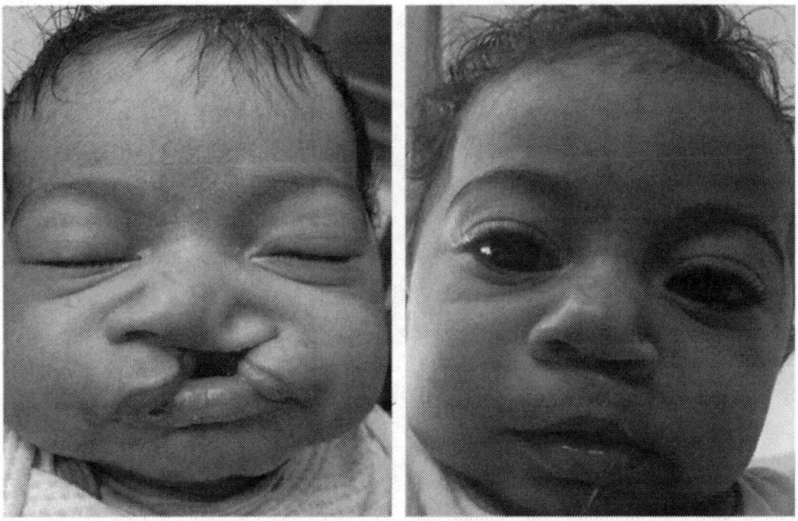

Before and after surgery for cleft lip and palate.

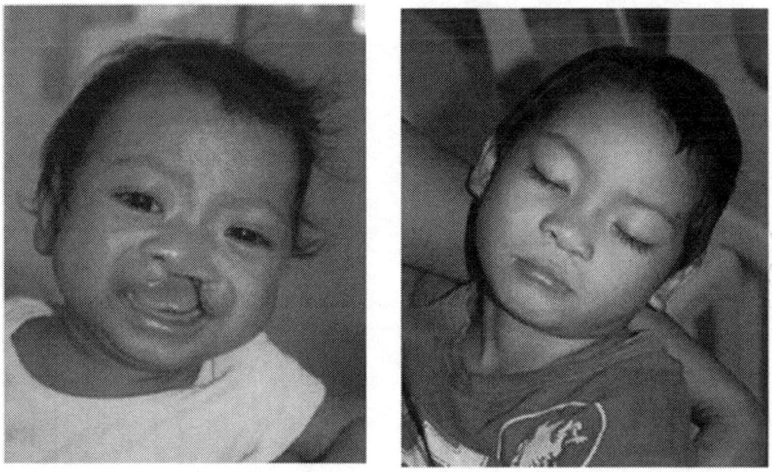

Before and after surgery for cleft lip.

Each cleft lip or palate that John repaired was truly a miracle. Looking at the two children above, imagine what kind of life awaited them if they had to live with such disfigurement.

After evaluating Fetu, John decided to do surgery on him. Because he was already 40 years old, the tissues were less plastic and harder to work with, but John was confident he could help him.

The surgery took over two hours, and everything went well. A dentist was present to help realign Fetu's teeth.

A year later, I got an email from John saying that Fetu was doing well and had found a wife, as well as a better job working as a gardener at one of the hotels in Apia.

Chapter 14
Robert Louis Stevenson

SATURDAY MORNING, Dr. Gosh and I decided to visit the Robert Louis Stevenson Museum. We took a taxi from our hotel to Vailima, where the museum was located. Vailima beer was also named after the village.

The museum sat on top of a hill. The taxi dropped us off at the entrance by the road, an easy five-minute stroll from the main house. The road leading to it was lined with tall, beautiful royal palm trees. The house had two stories, which I learned was the first two-story house ever built in Samoa.

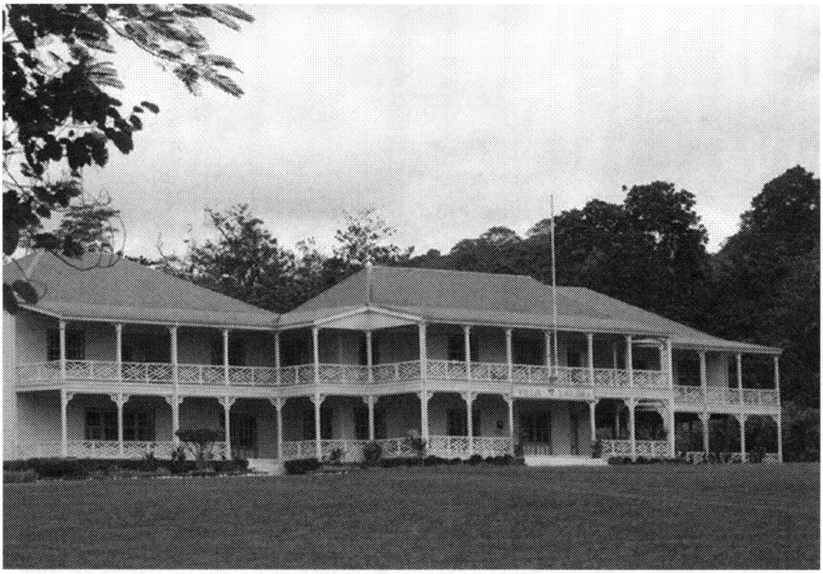

The Robert Louis Stevenson Museum at Vailima, Samoa.

When it was completed, the big house had five bedrooms, a library, a ballroom large enough to accommodate 100 dancers, and the only fireplace in Samoa. The Stevensons shipped 72 tons of furniture from England, all of which was hauled the 5 km (3 miles) from Apia on sleds pulled by bullocks. A piano sat in one corner of the great hall, in a glass case to protect it from Samoa's humidity. Among their possessions were a Rodin nude presented to Stevenson by the sculptor himself, a damask tablecloth from Queen Victoria, and a sugar bowl used by both Robert Burns and Sir Walter Scott, another writer from Scotland.

Admission was about $10 U.S., and the young woman who was our guide did an excellent job of explaining the different artifacts in the museum as well the life stories of the people who lived there. In the center of the living room, roped off, was the skin of a large lion with its head on. Judging from the photos displayed, the house was left as it was lived in. I was impressed by how well kept the place was.

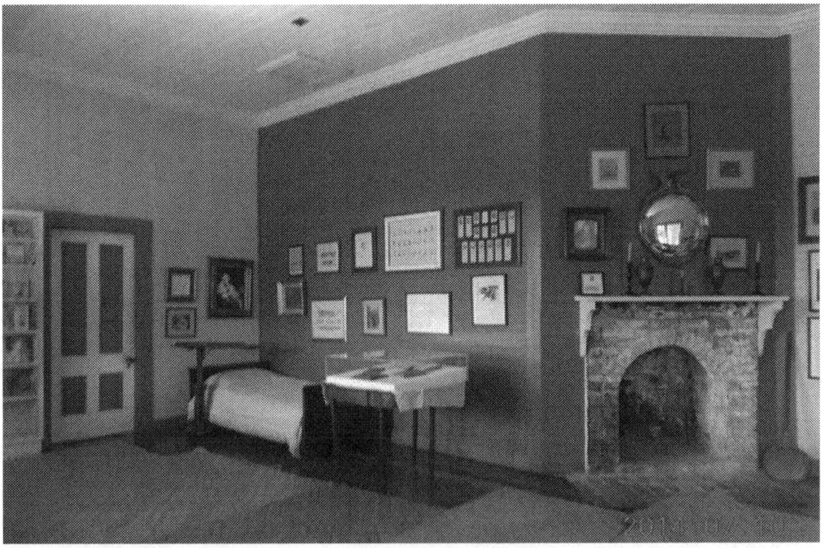

The bed in which Stevenson did much of his writing during his four years in Samoa.

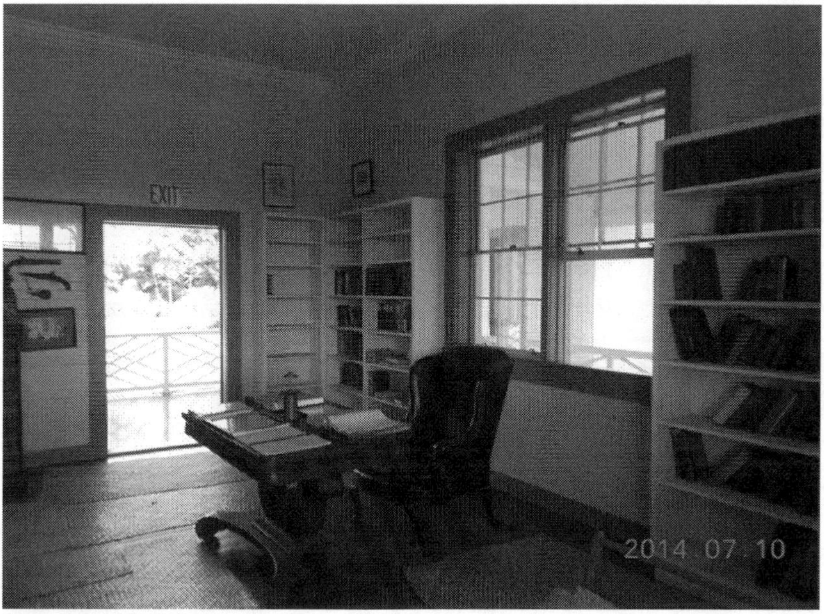

Stevenson's Library.

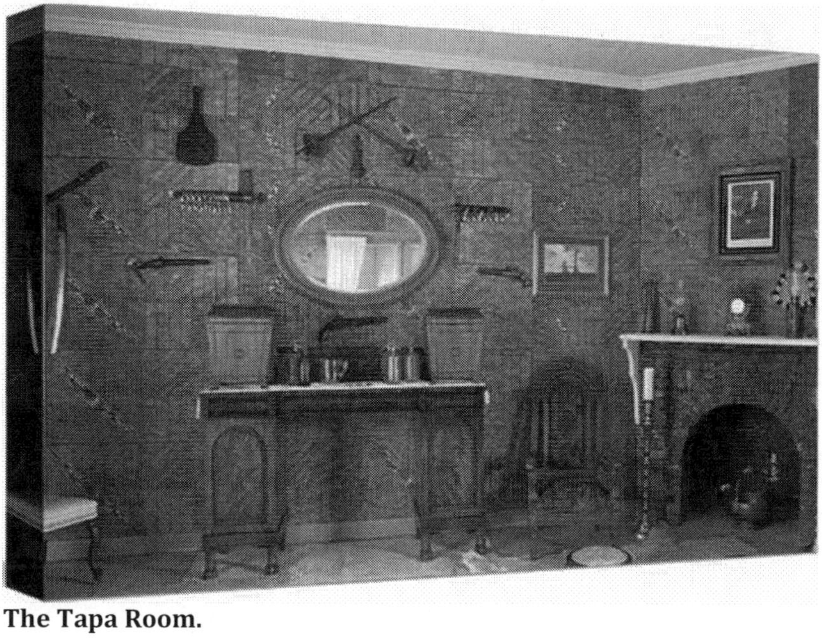

The Tapa Room.

After the tour of the house, Dr. Gosh and I decided to hike uphill to Stevenson's grave. It was a steep and difficult climb that took about half an hour. It had rained recently and the path was muddy and slippery most of the way. We often had to hang onto the branches of shrubs on either side of the path to keep from falling.

The trail was buried in a maze of fallen trees, so big and so close together that the hillside looked like a log jam. Their own weight had brought them crashing down, their roots pulling loose as frequent rains turned Samoa's volcanic soil to slippery muck.

A jumble of branches with leaves in various stages of withering lay on the path. There were tangles of exposed roots and gigantic trunks. There was enough space to wriggle under most of them, but with some, my only choice was to crawl over.

During Stevenson's life, there was no path at all, though he managed to climb to the top of Mt. Vaea and enjoy its magnificent view over green slopes running down to Apia, and the blue ocean beyond.

Stevenson had been one of my heroes because he was a great traveler and a prolific travel writer. I truly enjoyed reading his accounts of sailing around the South Pacific.

He was barely 40 when he and his family arrived in Samoa, but he was already world-famous thanks to *Treasure Island* and *The Strange Case of Dr. Jekyll and Mr. Hyde*, as well as travel books, essays and a myriad of poems.

Stevenson wrote a dozen more books in the four short years he lived there. He took sides in local politics, and was—and still is—much revered by the Samoan people. They called him *Tusitala*, the Teller of Tales.

As Dr. Gosh and I stood at Stevenson's grave, the heavy air coalesced into rain. By the time we got back to the trailhead, it was pelting down.

We walked back to the main road, bought a bottle of cold water at a grocery shack and drank half of it without stopping to breathe. Then we flagged down one of the island's brightly painted buses—this one converted from an old school bus—and rode it into central Apia and trudged back to the Annabelle Inn.

In the seventh grade in Malaysia, one of the books we had to read was *Treasure Island*. Even though it was only 104 pages, I found the reading difficult because of the way it was written in 1883, and I was unfamiliar with some of the word usage. But I liked story and greatly admired the author. Later, in college, I had to read *Dr. Jekyll and Mr. Hyde*, which I found a lot easier to read.

When I went to Hawaii for university, I would sometimes have dinner at the Waioli Tea Room in Manoa Valley not far from campus. I learned that the facility had been owned by the Salvation Army, and someone told me that Stevenson had stayed there before he went on to Samoa. The well that used to provide water for the building had a small sign that read "Robert Louis Stevenson was here." It was a small sign that didn't look very official, and I often doubted if he really stayed there, as I couldn't find any information about it in my research. He spent five months in Hawaii, but had stayed initially with his friend, Henry Poor, and later rented the house next door.

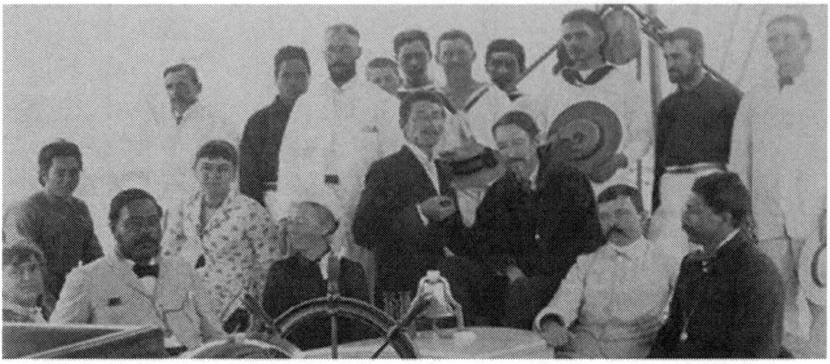

Sailing with friends around Waikiki. Stevenson is in the front row, third from the right, with a mustache and wearing a black coat.

While he was in Hawaii, Stevenson was presented to King Kalakaua at the Iolani Palace, where a feast was held in his honor. He met the king's sister, Princess Likelike, her husband, Edinburgh-born Archibald Cleghorn, and their daughter and heir to the Hawaiian throne, 13-year-old Princess Ka'iulani. Stevenson was enchanted by the young princess and struck up a playful, paternalistic friendship with her.

Princess Ka'iulani was set to leave Hawaii to be educated in England after traveling to Scotland and across Europe. Before her departure, Stevenson wrote *The Island Rose.*

Forth from her land to mine she goes,
The island maid, the island rose,
Light of heart and bright of face:
The daughter of a double race.
Her islands here, in Southern sun,
Shall mourn their Kaiulani gone,
And I, in her dear banyan shade,
Look vainly for my little maid.
But our Scots islands far away
Shall glitter with unwonted day,
And cast for once their tempests by
To smile in Kaiulani's eye.

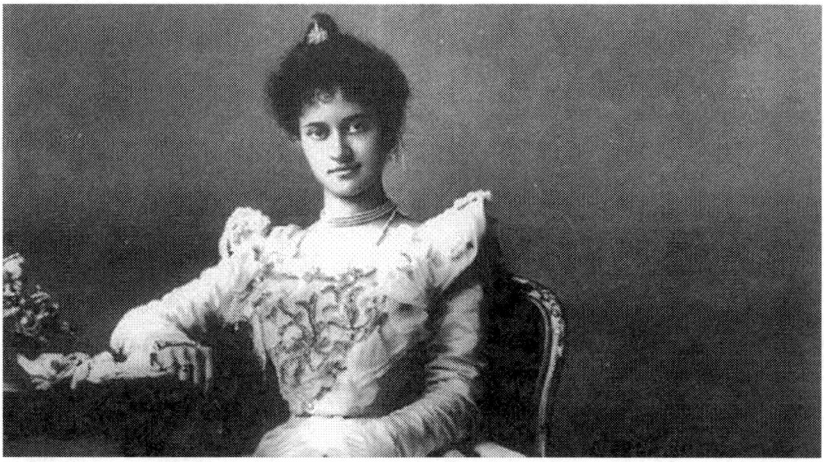

Princess Kaiulani.

I thought it was such a beautiful poem, and I too was enchanted by the princess. During my first year at the University of Hawaii, I was invited to a prom at the Sacred Heart High School in Honolulu. It was held at the Princess Ka'iulani Hotel in Waikiki. In the lobby was a large portrait of her. I was so impressed by how regal she looked and imagined how she conducted herself at the court of King Kalakaua, her uncle. I later read what I could about her and was sad to learn that she died at age 24 of pneumonia.

Having read most of Robert Louis Stevenson's books and discovering his Hawaii connection, I was fascinated by what a short but exciting life he lived. As an avid traveler myself, I was in awe of how widely he traveled at a time when traveling wasn't at all easy.

He'd been a sickly boy, and illness plagued him into his adult life and left him extremely thin. He was suspected to have tuberculosis, but more recent views are that it was bronchiectasis or even sarcoidosis. I was impressed that he didn't let it stop him from writing or exploring the world.

He began studying engineering at the University of Edinburgh in 1867, but lacked enthusiasm for it and mainly put his energy into avoiding lectures. He switched to studying law, but he never practiced. He was more interested in travel and writing. One of his journeys was a canoe voyage in Belgium and France.

In September of 1876, he met Indianapolis-born Fanny Van de Grift Osbourne (1840–1914). She had married at age 17 and had two children, Isobel ("Belle") and Lloyd, eventually separating from her husband as a result of his infidelities. When Stevenson met her, she was living in France, where she and Belle studied art and she had become a magazine short-story writer of recognized ability.

Stevenson then traveled overland by train from New York City to California. He later wrote about the experience in *The Amateur Emigrant*. The long overland journey took a toll on him and he got very sick.

By December 1879, Stevenson had recovered his health enough to continue to San Francisco.

In May 1880, he and Fanny were married. The couple, along with Fanny's son Lloyd, traveled to Napa Valley and spent the summer at an abandoned mining camp on Mount Saint Helena (now called the Robert Louis Stevenson State Park). He wrote about this experience in *The Silverado Squatters*.

For the next several years, the Stevensons shuttled back and forth between Scotland and the Continent, finally settling in 1884 in the English seaside town of Bournemouth in Dorset.

Although he was in ill health and largely bedridden, Stevenson wrote the bulk of his most popular work during his time in Dorset: *Treasure Island, Kidnapped, The Strange Case of Dr. Jekyll and Mr. Hyde* and *The Black Arrow: A Tale of the Two Roses.*

After his father died in 1887, Stevenson decided to follow his physician's advice and try a complete change of climate. The family, including Stevenson's mother, headed for Colorado, but after landing in New York, they decided to spend the winter in the Adirondacks at Saranac Lake, at a cottage now known as Stevenson Cottage. During an intensely cold winter, Stevenson wrote some of his best essays, including *Pulvis et Umbra*. He also began *The Master of Ballantrae* and planned a cruise to the southern Pacific Ocean for the following summer.

After their time in Hawaii, in December 1889, Stevenson and his extended family arrived at the port of Apia in the Samoan islands, and there he and Fanny decided to settle. In January 1890, they purchased 314¼ acres at Vailima, some miles inland from Apia, on which they built their house—now the museum Dr. Gosh and I visited.

While Fanny set about managing and working the estate, Stevenson took the native name Tusitala and began collecting local stories. His first work of literature in Samoan was *The Bottle Imp*.

The story centers around a bottle in which an imp, a little demon, lives. The imp grants the bottle owner's every wish, but anybody who still has the bottle when they die is cursed to eternal punishment in Hell.

Stevenson's health improved greatly in the warm climate of Samoa, and he was immensely pleased with his decision to move there.

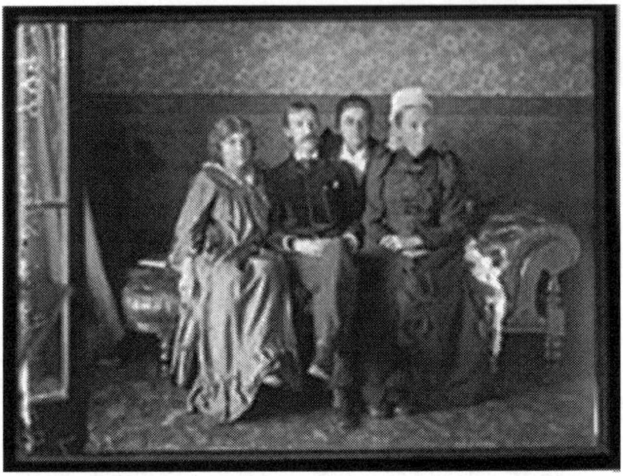

From left to right: Stevenson's wife Fanny, Stevenson, Fanny's son Lloyd and Stevenson's mother, Margaret, in Vailima, Samoa, c. 1892.

I read with interest some of his daily accounts:

March 19th 1891. Before the sun rises, at 5:45 or 5:50, Paul brings me tea, bread, and a couple of eggs; and by about six I am at work. I work in bed—my bed is of mats, no mattress, sheets, or filth—mats, a pillow, and a blanket—and put in some three hours. It was 9:05 this morning when I set off to the stream-side to my weeding; where I toiled, manuring the ground with the best enricher, human sweat, till the conch-shell was blown from our verandah at 10:30.

He continued to write, sending his work back to America and Europe by the steamer services. In this way, he earned enough to keep them in a reasonable financial position and to support the establishment and hangers-on.

Immersing himself in the islands' culture, and learning to love and respect the Polynesian people, Stevenson was distressed by how the Europeans were exploiting the islands. He soon felt it was his duty to warn the Samoan people of the motives of these Europeans, citing what they had done to the kingdom of Hawaii.

The rival great powers were Britain, Germany and the United States, whose warships were a common sight in Samoan harbors. Stevenson understood that, as in the Scottish Highlands, an indigenous clan society was unprepared for the arrival of foreigners who played upon its existing rivalries and divisions. As the external pressures upon Samoan society grew, tensions soon developed into several inter-clan wars.

In 1892, Stevenson wrote *A Footnote to History: Eight Years of Trouble in Samoa*, a detailed chronicle of the rivalries between the great powers and the first Samoan Civil War.

Stevenson was alarmed above all by what he perceived as the Samoans' economic innocence. In 1894, just months before his death, he addressed the island chiefs:

There is but one way to defend Samoa. Hear it before it is too late. It is to make roads, and gardens, and care for your trees, and sell their produce wisely, and, in one word, to occupy and use your country.... if you do not occupy and use your country, others will. It will not continue to be yours or your children's, if you occupy it for nothing. You and your children will in that case be cast out into outer darkness....

Five years after Stevenson's death, the Samoan Islands were partitioned between Germany and the United States.

On December 3rd, 1894, Stevenson was talking to his wife and straining to open a bottle of wine when he suddenly asked, "What's that?" and then, "Does my face look strange?" and collapsed. He died within a few hours, probably of a cerebral hemorrhage. He was 44 years old. The Samoans insisted on surrounding his body with a watch-guard during the night and then carried him on their shoulders to nearby Mount Vaea, where they buried him in a spot overlooking the sea.

Stevenson had always wanted his Requiem inscribed on his tomb:

Under the wide and starry sky,
Dig the grave and let me lie.
Glad did I live and gladly die,
And I laid me down with a will.
This be the verse you grave for me:
Here he lies where he longed to be;
Home is the sailor, home from sea,
And the hunter home from the hill.

Stevenson was loved by the Samoans, and his tombstone epigraph was translated to a Samoan song of grief.

Fanny died in California in 1914, and her ashes were brought back to Vailima and buried at the foot of her husband's grave. Her Samoan name, Aolele, is engraved on a bronze plaque.

Vailima eventually became the property of the Samoan Government, and for many years, Samoa's head of state lived in the house. It was the scene of many formal functions and entertainments until hurricanes severely damaged the mansion in 1990 and 1991.

When repairs began, it was decided that Vailima should be turned into a museum. Since then, an extraordinary renovation has returned it to the state it was in when Stevenson lived there.

A celebrity in his own time, Stevenson was admired by many other writers, including Marcel Proust, Arthur Conan Doyle, Henry James, Ernest Hemingway, Rudyard Kipling, Jack London and Vladimir Nabokov.

For much of the 20th century he was seen as a second-class writer, relegated to children's literature and horror genres; but today his works are generally acclaimed. The late 20th century saw a re-evaluation of Stevenson as an artist of great range and insight, a literary theorist, an essayist and social critic, a witness to the colonial history of the Pacific Islands and a humanist. He has remained popular worldwide, and in 2018 was ranked just behind Charles Dickens as the 26th most translated author in the world.

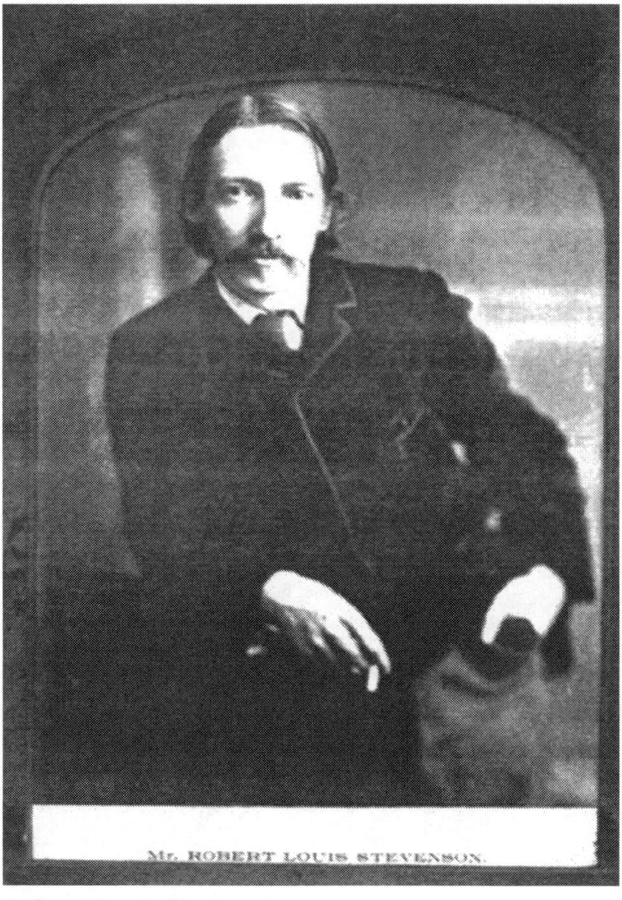

Robert Louis Stevenson.

Chapter 15

Chinese in Samoa

As I MET PEOPLE in both Samoa and American Samoa, I came across several doctors with Chinese surnames. They all knew that they had either a Chinese grandfather or great-grandfather.

It's been estimated that 30% of the residents of Samoa have a degree of Chinese heritage. Because of the inclusive nature of Samoan society, most of them are considered totally Samoan. It's only through surnames like Ah Mu, Ah Wong, Ah Kan, etc. that they know they must have descended from a Chinese ancestor two or three generations ago.

In 1880, the King of Samoa, Susuga Malietoa Laupepa, had declared that no further Chinese would be permitted to settle in Samoa. Apparently the consuls representing the European settlers put pressure on Malietoa Laupepa to issue the decree, most likely because they feared and resented the commercial success most early Chinese settlers had achieved. Despite the king's declaration, Malietoa Laupepa's government doesn't seem to have enforced it, as Chinese free settlers continued to arrive in Samoa.

The early 1900s saw an influx of plantation workers from China. In a 2015 talk on the history of the Chinese in Samoa, Samoan Attorney General, Tuatagaloa Aumua Ming Leung Wai, explained the early twentieth-century need for these foreign workers:

Samoan people were comfortable with their lifestyle of subsistence living so did not want to work in the commercial plantations owned by the Europeans. Another contemporary of the time said that it was "impossible for the Samoan to fit into the role of a steady plantation workman because he has no conception of western industrial life". This meant that the European owners of these plantations had to look outside of Samoa for labour.

The German plantation owners found that the Chinese were extremely reliable workers and began bringing them into Samoa.

Chinese emigration was more out of necessity than the desire to leave the land of their fathers. By the end of the 19th century, conditions in China were so grave that many people were starving, and the desire to migrate had become almost an obsession in order to survive. Many Chinese men dreamed of amassing huge fortunes in the gold mines and plantations of newly developed colonies. Those who ended up in the Pacific did so mainly through the indentured labor system.

Indentured labor is a system in which a person who takes out a loan agrees to work without salary for the lender for a specific number of years—usually from three to five. Historically, it's been used to pay the cost of the person's transportation to job locations all over the world.

According to official records, about 7,000 Chinese immigrated to Samoa under the dreaded indentured labor system. Many of these men had little or no idea what sort of a place Samoa was. Most of them were illiterate and signed the agreement through a broker, who often acted as the witness as well, without understanding it.

The following is an example of a contract for a Chinese indentured laborer.

0131

合同格式

立合同人工主　　代理人　工人

今將兩家所訂作工合同開列於後

一該工人定本日起程前往薩摩地方赴上開工主指定之園地作工

二該工人每逢作工之日操作不過十點鐘

三該工主每月應給工人辛金　員

四該工人已經支領上期銀　員須由工錢扣回每月　員

五凡遇華人放假日期工人不必操作

六工人所有伙食住所醫藥均由工主出資支理供給

七工人如有不肯作工應聽工主計算日期扣除工錢其有自恢因而患病
不能作工者亦照此辦理工主與工人如有因此或因別事爭執均可
稟赴地方官稟明聽候核斷

八工人倘若未蒙監管頭人允准不得擅離園地

九合同期限三年爲滿係由工人到薩摩地方之日起算

十合同期滿工人有欲回華者自必資遣返國

十一彼此有因合同詞意爭執者應以德文爲準

上開各款兩家均已閱悉應允玆特各自簽名於下以昭信實

工人簽名

主工簽名

證人簽名

This contract reads vertically from right to left, and is written in simple Chinese. The first column lists the name of the laborer, the employer and the broker. The second column explains that the contract was signed with mutual agreement.

The agreement has 11 conditions:

1. (Date) to begin work at (Name of the) plantation.
2. Work should not exceed 10 hours a day.
3. The monthly wages would be ___ German Marks. Typically, the wages for a month were 10 marks (about $2.40 US at the time).
4. Since the worker has already been paid ____, wages will be deducted for ___(amount of time).
5. No work on Chinese holidays, such as New Year, Mid-autumn Festival plus 8 other holidays.
6. Room and board and medical expenses will be paid by the employer.
7. If the worker refuses to work, pay will be deducted accordingly. If a worker cannot work because of illness, the local authority will decide such a claim. If the worker has a conflict with the employer, local officials will rule on such conflicts.
8. Without permission of the employer, the worker cannot leave the plantation.
9. The contract is for 3 years, beginning on the day the worker arrives in Samoa.
10. When the contract is up, if the worker wishes to return to China, he will pay his own way.
11. If there is any conflict between the employer and worker, the language to resolve the dispute will be in German.

Then the last three columns are the signature of the worker, employer and a witness.

The following table shows the names of the ships that brought laborers to Apia. It contains the date of arrival of each of the ship and the number of laborers it carried.

From 1903 to 1934, a total of 6,984 Chinese laborers were brought to Apia. It's also possible that other Chinese arrived in Samoa on other ships.

This table only provides information from 1903 on. Chinese had arrived in Samoa long before this.

批数	抵达阿皮亚日期	船名	每船人数	累计人数
1	1903.04.28	德西马号	289	289
2	1905.05.30	前进号	528	817
3	1906.07.22	赫尔斯坦号	575	1392
4	1908.06.10	前进号	251	1743
5	1909.11.28	麦西尔德号	535	2278
6	1911.12.28	帕克拉克号	551	2829
7	1913.05.08	密歇尔·杰普森号	1039	3868
8	1920.08.09	哈尔蒂斯号	502	4370
9	1921.10.07	爱斯科特号	959	5329
10	1925.04.12	新麦西尔德号	280	5609
11	1926.08.16	海庆号	180	5789
12	1928.04.14	海洋号	456	6245
13	1930.05.08	阿波伊号	251	6496
14	1931.09.08	阿波伊号	207	6703
15	1934.07.27	赛斯坦号	281	6984

Arrival date **Vessel name** **# of workers**

The last column is the total number of workers arrived in Apia.

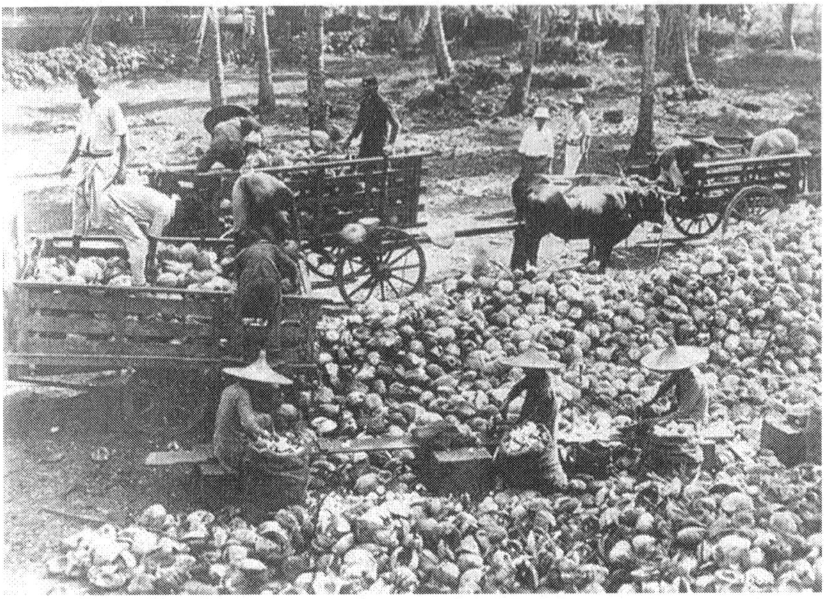

Chinese men working on a coconut planation, circa 1910.

Sometimes the Chinese laborers were treated poorly, and flogging was routine. The plantation owners thought they were being humane by limiting the flogging to once a week at a maximum of 20 lashers per person! According to Tuatagaloa Aumua Ming Leung Wai:

> *Flogging could result from: "hiding, laziness, running away, disobedience, insulting behavior, breaking the curfew and even for not bowing low enough in respect of their masters."*
> *....[But] despite the hardships faced by the Chinese laborers, they were hard workers and were described as "the most reliable and trustworthy labor yet available" by the weekly German language newspaper* Samoanische Zeitung.

World War I was not going well for Germany, and on August 29th, 1914, New Zealand's Expeditionary force arrived in Samoa and replaced the German Administration.

This new military administration from New Zealand, in light of the poor treatment of the Chinese laborers and in order to protect them, decreed that the workers should return to China. Soon, wholesale repatriation of the Chinese laborers began. Between 1914 and 1918, three major repatriations took place, which reduced the Chinese labor force in Samoa to about 832.

The labor shortage had a negative effect on the agriculture industry in Samoa and pushed many plantation owners toward bankruptcy. The situation was exacerbated by the canker disease on the cocoa plantations and the rhinoceros beetle infestation on the coconut plantations. The angry planters demanded the return of Chinese laborers.

Before long, wholesale repatriations stopped and some of the Chinese laborers who were still in Samoa were re-hired.

While some were happy to return to China, others wanted to remain in Samoa, especially those who had married locals and had children. However, repatriation of the Chinese was still forced, probably motivated by fears that the Chinese would dominate Samoan businesses, given their proven reputation as industrious, hardworking and economically driven.

It was a sad chapter in Samoa's long history of inclusion, as the forcible repatriation separated families. In 1916, about 100 Chinese laborers were married to or in relationships with Samoan women, with a combined total of 108 Chinese-Samoan children. By 1930, the number of Samoans with Chinese heritage had risen to between 1,000 and 1,500. Despite this, the New Zealand Administration maintained its policy of returning laborers to China.

Most Samoan-Chinese were unable to locate or trace their Chinese families, and many of them suffered greatly trying to live in a country they no longer knew.

As Tuatagaloa Aumua Ming Leung Wai explains:

> *Generally, only the surnames of Chinese laborers were used when they were converted into English.... Converting them back to Chinese was therefore a problem if the first name is not known. No proper records relating to their identification could be found. It also didn't help that the laborers were usually referred to by numbers instead of their names, eg Yue Yiek was known as "Coolie No. 398". Employment contracts and letters exchanged between Government officials and employers mostly referred to the Chinese laborers by their Coolie numbers.*

In addition to forceful repatriation, the Chinese laborers also experienced racism from some Europeans who considered them sub-human. At one point, during the German administration, laws were passed to keep Chinese laborers from moving about too freely and to keep Samoan women off the plantations.

When New Zealand took over the administration of Samoa, further laws were passed aimed at preventing Chinese men and Samoan women from forming relationships. For example, a proclamation issued in 1917 prohibited Chinese indentured laborers from entering any Samoan's house. It was also an offence for a Samoan to allow a Chinese laborer onto his premises. Anyone breaking these laws was subject to a fine of up to five pounds or hard-labor imprisonment for up to six weeks. A further proclamation forbade Samoan women to visit the labor quarters.

New Zealand passed another law in 1921 that prohibited Chinese indentured laborers from marrying Samoan women. The penalty for breaking the law was a fine of 20 pounds or imprisonment for six months. According to the *Pacific Islands Monthly* (July 15th, 1939), 34 Chinese men and their wives were in jail for breaching the law at the time, the men serving three months, and the women serving three days.

These discriminatory legislations reflected the racist attitude of some of the influential Europeans at the time towards the Chinese. Such racism was usually veiled in the guise of keeping the Samoan race pure. There were fears that the Chinese would contaminate the Samoan race. However, it was claimed that unions between Samoans and Europeans were accepted because the children from these unions were of "fair skinned and of Aryan stock". (Tuatagaloa Aumua Ming Leung Wai)

Unfortunately, some Samoans also showed anti-Chinese attitudes, following the example set by European sentiments. The Samoan central native administration issued a decree ordering Samoan women to leave their Chinese husbands and return to their Samoan families. Subsequently, Samoan villages passed regulations that prohibited cohabitation between Chinese laborers and Samoan women.

Tuatagaloa Aumua Ming Leung Wai explains further:

> *This was no surprise given the statements made by the first head of the New Zealand military administration in Samoa that the Chinese were "inferior" and were a threat to the racial purity of Samoa. In addition, he added that Samoans disliked the Chinese. However, his successor Tate disputed this. Tate stated that "The Samoan women recognise the Chinese as better husbands than the Samoan men." In fact, before the arrival of the Europeans, mixed marriages were accepted, and at times, valued by the Samoan culture.*

***

I met a G.P. in Samoa whose last name was Ah-Ching. When he discovered I was Chinese, he asked me if I knew what his last name meant in Chinese. He said his grandfather's full name was Ah Ching Sin San.

I answered that the name Ching, Chen or Chan 陳 is one of the most common Chinese surnames, numbering in the millions, and that Ah doesn't really mean anything. Almost all Chinese men who arrived in Samoa had Ah added to their surname because it was easier for Westerners and Samoans to pronounce them as two-syllable names rather than a single syllable. Adding Ah to the surname is a common way to address another Chinese, a sort of nickname.

Sin San means Mister. So, Ah Ching Sin San simply means Mr. Ching. It would be little help to Dr. Ah-Ching in tracing his grandfather's roots in China.

He said his grandfather, who had married a Samoan woman, never spoke about China so the family had no idea where he came from.

I met another doctor, Dr. Nathan Chong, whose grandfather Foo Chong arrived in Samoa as an indentured laborer. After working on a coconut plantation for a few years, he married a Samoan woman and was able to get a piece of land. He was given a Samoan name, Papaseea. Foo Chong worked hard on his land and grew many different types of Chinese vegetables, which the Samoans loved. He became very successful.

Nathan remembered his grandpa fondly. Foo Chong taught him to work hard and tried to teach him Chinese, but had passed away when Nathan was just nine years old. Because of his grandfather's financial success, Nathan was able to attend medical school in Fiji.

He still could say a few words in Chinese. From his accent, I decided that his grandpa must have come from the Toishan area, not far from Guangzhou and Hong Kong. The dialect is similar to the Cantonese in Hong Kong but with a regional accent.

In addition to explaining the general history of the Chinese community in Samoa, Tuatagaloa Aumua Ming Leung Wai also spoke about his own Chinese heritage during his 2015 lecture.

His great-grandfather Leung Wai (a.k.a. Ah Wai or Avai) was from Toishan, in Guangdong Province in southern China. He was born on October 12, 1886. One week after he got married, he left China for Samoa, around the age of 24.

Leung Wai worked very hard and saved enough money to start his own business. He became quite successful and had various businesses such as a laundry, butchery, plantations, farms, restaurants and taxis.

Like many Chinese men, in spite of being married in China, he took on a Samoan wife, a woman named Lealofi-o-Amoa Luafalealii Falenaoti Segi from the island of Savaii.

Leung Wai's eldest son Ming (Tuatagaloa Aumua's grandfather, whom he was named after) was sent to China at age eight for his education. Ming was born in 1918 in Saasaai, Savaii. He went to China around 1926 and stayed with Leung Wai's Chinese wife, who raised him as her own.

Ming later married a Chinese woman from Toishan in Guangdong, China named Hung Lock. She later adopted the Western name Hana. She was Tuatagaloa Aumua's grandmother. Before they were married, Hana's family had many questions for Ming, as he (who was half-Samoan) was tall and had brown skin. This was unusual because the Chinese in Southern China were fairer skinned and much shorter than most Samoans.

Ming and Hana had five children. The hardship caused by the Japanese occupation of China (1937 –1945) resulted in the deaths of their four eldest children. Tuatagaloa Aumua's grandmother Hana used to tell him how they would hide in the bushes to avoid the Japanese soldiers and eat grass to survive, as there was no food.

Ming and Hana's only surviving child was Tuatagaloa Aumua's father, Bee Leung Wai.

Ming, Hana and Bee managed to leave China in 1950 and travel to Samoa by ship via Sydney, Australia. Money to pay for their passage was sent over by Tuatagaloa Aumua's great-grandfather, Leung Wai.

Bee Leung Wai married Taituuga Kuinivia Aumua, and their son, Tuatagaloa Aumua Ming Leung Wai, became a prominent Samoan and later, the Attorney General of the country.

In his talk, Tuatagaloa Aumua Ming Leung Wai also tells the story of another Chinese immigrant:

> *Another Chinese free settler who came to Samoa in the first wave of Chinese migration was Ah Mu. He came around 1875. He was "adopted" by British sailors at a very young age when their vessel called into one of the Chinese ports. When he got tired of travelling with the British navy he decided to settle in Samoa. He started a carting and transporting business before expanding into other areas such as repairing wheels, shoeing horses, dairy, and a Ford car dealership.*
> *....One of Ah Mu's grandsons (M. Ah Mu) fought in World War 1 and had served in France and Palestine. Some descendants of Ah Mu have used "Rivers" as their surname. There is a prestigious private primary school called "Ah Mu Academy" located at Pesega named after this famous early Chinese settler. Constance Tafua-Rivers, one of the senior lawyers in my Office is a descendant of Ah Mu. One of Ah Mu's well-known descendants is Hon. Hans Joe Keil who was a former Cabinet Minister and is a successful businessman.*

Again, Samoan society is traditionally a very inclusive one. Inter-marriage between races is generally accepted. This is why the Chinese who migrated to Samoa were able to assimilate with ease into the Samoan culture, in spite of efforts made by some Europeans to stop it.

Chapter 16

German-Samoans

MANY OF THE IMPORTANT PEOPLE I'VE MET in Samoa seem to have German names, and I've been fascinated by how much influence the Germans had on the country.

When I was in private practice in California, I became friends with Dr. Frederick Uhle, an internist, whose grandfather came from Germany and whose mother was the post mistress of American Samoa. My good friend John's father was German or part German, and the young doctor, Robert Schultz, who I met at the hospital was also part German. A patient I saw at the eye clinic, who owned all the radio stations in Samoa, had a German name and looked more German than Samoan. The largest hardware store in Apia was owned by a man with a German name, and I noticed that many of the politicians also had German names.

The period of German rule in Samoa spanned only 1900–1914, but German influence started much earlier than that. At the time of the German occupation, Samoa was already a thriving place with many of the locals educated in German.

Compared to other European colonial powers, Germany had done a good job trying to develop Samoa and treated the people fairly. Unlike other colonies, such as Fiji, Samoa doesn't have a racial problem resulting from the introduction of foreign laborers. Fiji is now a country divided between the natives and the Indians who were brought to the island with their families to work on the sugar plantations. In Samoa, the laborers Germany brought in were small in number and only men. As discussed in the previous chapter, most of these laborers were Chinese men who ended up marrying Samoan women. Their descendants became Samoan citizens.

The German language carried a degree of prestige in Samoa, and a large number of Samoans made efforts to learn it; although, ironically, many native German speakers were known to prefer English. The colonial dialect that developed in Samoa drew words from both English and Samoan and wasn't fully comprehensible to other Germans speakers. It was spoken in most homes of mixed German-Samoan families.

Some families who had the means sent their sons to Germany for higher education.

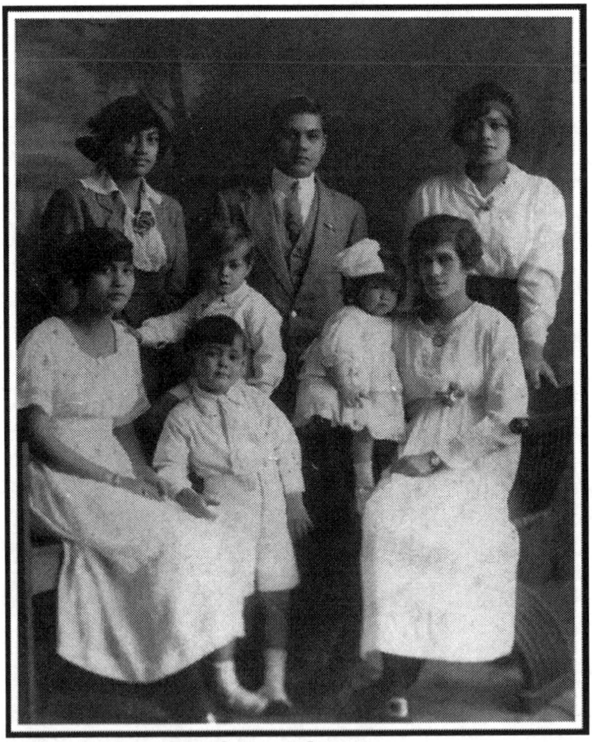

German-Samoan descendants.

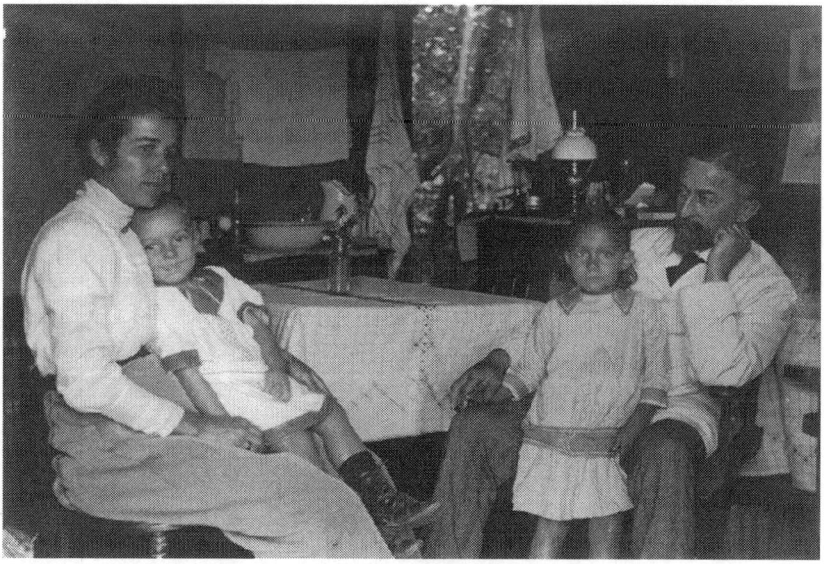

A German man with his Samoan wife and children.

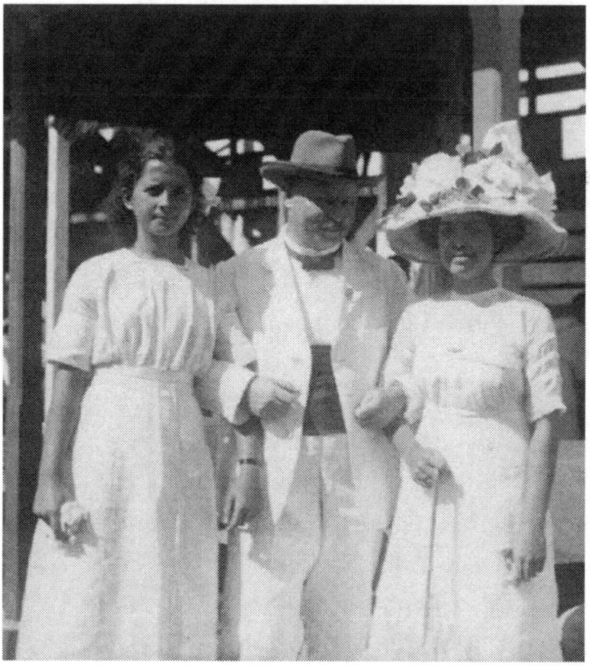

A German man with his Samoan wife and daughter.

As I researched the history of the Germans in Samoa, a few prominent Samoan citizens with German heritage stood out to me.

The Telefoni Retzlaff Family

The Honorable Misa Telefoni Retzlaff, as he is addressed, has been active in Samoan politics for many years. He was also the Deputy Leader of the Human Rights Protection Party (HRPP). His responsibilities included membership in the European Union (EU) and World Trade Organization (WTO).

He was Attorney General of Samoa from 1986–1988 and had been a Member of Parliament since 1988 and a Minister of State since 1992, as well as serving in many other positions.

Retzlaff's grandfather, Erich Retzlaff, was born in Stettin, which is now a part of Poland and known as Szczecin. Their family owned a small farm on the city's outskirts.

His elder brother, Hermann Retzlaff, inherited the farm, so in spite of his love for farming, Erich reluctantly took a position at the Post Office and moved to Berlin. His job involved putting up telephone lines and connecting telephones.

In 1906, he arrived in Samoa aboard the SS Holstein with 30 telephones in tow, along with 75 Chinese workers from the German colony in Guangzhou, China.

He became known universally by the Samoans as Telefoni because of his work as a telephone installer, and to this day the family is still known as the Telefoni Family in Samoa.

Erich Retzlaff met and fell in love with Elizabeth Purcell, a woman of Irish-Samoan ancestry, and they married in 1913. Their son, Hermann Paul Retzlaff, was born on March 23rd, 1914. He later married Piliopo Joyce Rosabel Nelson. These were Misa Telefoni Retzlaff's parents.

Misa was born Hermann Theodor Retzlaff on May 21st, 1952 in Apia; but in Samoa, he was generally known as Misa Telefoni Retzlaff.

Misa has three *matai* (chief) titles: Misa from Matautu Falelatai—1984; Lesamatauanu'u from Malaela Aleipata—1986; and Tugaga from Faletagaloa Safune—1987.

The Keil Family

Another prominent Samoan with a German name is the Honorable Hans Joachim Keil III, the Pacific Region's lead negotiator of the Economic Partnership Agreement (EPA) with the European Union (EU).

His grandfather, Hans Joachim Keil I, was born on April 20th, 1864 in Magdeburg, Prussia, Germany. At age 29, he met and married Johanna Wilhelmine Elise Ronnecke, nee Henze.

In 1903, he and Elise arrived in Samoa on a steam ship. They had one son, and then Elise sadly passed away in 1908.

In 1909, Hans, at 45 years of age, married Daisy Ah Mu, a young woman from a prominent Chinese-Samoan family, aged 17. The couple had many children together. In 1948, Hans Joachim Keil I passed away.

Wilhelm Viktor Albert Keil, born in 1923, was the seventh Son of Hans Joachim Keil I and Daisy Ah Mu. He became the Honorary German Consul in Samoa for over 15 years, until his retirement in 2000.

The Honorable Hans Joachim Keil III is Wilhelm's second of seven sons. He has been a Member of Parliament (MP) since 1988, and a Minister of State for over 10 years, serving in the departments of Shipping, Transport, Tourism, Trade Commerce and Industry, and Labor.

He has served in the U.S. Air Force and has been a commercial airline pilot. He is also prominent in many Samoan businesses, owning a McDonald's Restaurant and the TV3 Television Broadcasting Station, and holding large shares in Hellaby Meats Ltd. and Lotto Samoa.

The descendants of Hans Joachim Keil I and Daisy Ah Mu number in the thousands today.

The Schmidt Family

Yet another prominent Samoan is the Honorable Deputy Speaker La'auli Leuatea Schmidt.

His great-great-grandfather, Albert Kurt von Schmidt, born in 1848, was from Hamburg, Germany. The family eventually dropped the "von" and began using Schmidt as their surname.

Albert Schmidt married Serah Clara Smith from Safotu Savaii (her father was from Vermont, USA, and her mother was Samoan) in 1872. La'auli Leuatea's great-grandfather, Bismarck Schmidt, was born in 1903. He later married Utu Taofinu'u Peseta Solia, and she gave birth to La'auli Leuatea's grandfather, Anselm Schmidt.

Anselm Schmidt married Filoi Tu'u, and the result of that union was nine children, the eighth of whom was La'auli Leuatea's father, Polataivao Asiata Fossie Schmidt.

The Honorable Polataivao Asiata Fossie Schmidt served in the Samoan government for over 30 years, including as Minister of State in Health, Lands, Commerce and Tourism. He married Puletiuatoa Fuimaono Ipuniuesea in 1958, and they had six children, the fourth of whom is the Honorable La'auli Leuatea Schmidt.

The Schmidt Family Reunion Commemorative Book contains genealogies that number Albert Kurt Schmidt's descendants in the thousands, spread throughout the world. Many have had distinguished careers, including a number of ordained Catholic nuns, priests and brothers, as well as pastors of other religious denominations.

In addition to these illustrious German-Samoans, I came across many more notable Samoans with German ancestry.

The late Dr. Hans Thieme's father was from Erfurt, and he was the first Samoan local to be made Director-General of Health. He was awarded the Samoa Order of Merit for his services to health by the Government in 1994.

Klaus Stunzner, Jr. is the current President of the Chamber of Commerce and is the grandson of Kurt Stunzner, born in Apia in 1906. The Stunzner family was originally from Dortmund.

The Von Reiches are a prominent business family in Samoa, and they trace their proud ancestry back to the city of Weimar in 1230.

Lynn Netzler is one of Apia's most prominent and successful businesswomen.

Muliufi Francis Hannemann had German ancestry and was from Samoa. He was elected twice as Mayor of Honolulu, in 2004 and 2008.

There were many more German names I came across in my research, and I was impressed to read about their long history in Samoa. I think it would be nearly impossible to document all the German or part-German families in Samoa.

As the Honorable Misa Telefoni Retzlaff himself states, "The German legacy in Samoa is an enduring legacy. It is both historical and contemporary because it is a story that continues still and has no end in sight."

Chapter 17

Strong Samoans

THE COUNTRY OF SAMOA has a population of only about 250,000 people. There are about 200,000 Samoans living in American Samoa and the continental U.S., but dozens of Samoans play in the NFL, American football's top league. The Samoan is 40 times more likely to play American football than any other ethnic group in America.

A good friend of mine, an American-born Chinese pharmacist and avid football fan, often lamented that he wasn't Samoan, or that his daughter hadn't married a Samoan. He wished he was a strong football player, or at least had one in the family.

There's no question that Samoans are born with an advantage of being built to play American football, where size and weight matter a great deal.

Why is it that so many Samoans are big and strong? The most commonly accepted theory proposed by anthropologists and evolution scientists is as follows:

Starting around 3,500 years ago, ancestors of Samoans began the arduous task of settling the 24 major island groups of Polynesia. This colonization process—one of the most extreme examples in all of human history—took possibly thousands of years to complete. They had to endure long voyages between islands and subsequently survive on those islands.

Pacific Islanders are a surprisingly new group of people, but they are a very separate ethnic group from east-Asian peoples like Malays or Filipinos. Originally, they lived on the island that is now Taiwan, and for some reason, around 1000 B.C., these Taiwanese aborigines left Asia and headed to Polynesia.

Looking at a map you can see that places like Samoa, Hawaii and New Zealand are very far from Taiwan, so the journey was incredibly perilous. Sailing across the enormous Pacific was considered dangerous to the rest of the world even when we were cruising across it in steamers and frigates, so the fact that these aborigines managed to get to Polynesia on outrigger canoes is truly amazing. It's likely that only the very strong and hardy were able to make it to their new homes in the Pacific.

It's believed that the travelers in the canoes most likely endured periods of starvation, and those who survived had an ability to store fat and conserve energy. This means that the more robust individuals had a survival advantage that was preserved in the descendants of these intrepid explorers.

A body that can conserve energy will gain more weight than one that doesn't, even if the calorie intake is the same. So, overall, Pacific Islanders are a naturally strong people, selected through thousands of years.

Once the first settlers landed in their new home, they continued living in tribal societies, which again favored the physically strong, as wars between villages were common, and survival was largely determined by how well a man could defend himself against other men. Most men would have to fight for their lives at some point. Those who beat the others survived to have children, and the great warriors were able to reproduce with many women. As a result, their descendants have large, strong bodies.

Some anthropologists have speculated that since small islands don't allow a lot of space for people to get away from a fight, over hundreds of years weaker Samoans were weeded out of the gene pool. Genes favoring a particular characteristic can take place in a smaller amount of time if the population is smaller to begin with. Darwin observed that the finches in the Galapagos, under certain conditions and usually on small islands, evolved in a much shorter time than finches elsewhere. He concluded that when environmental conditions are particularly severe, selection processes accelerate—an evolutionary phenomenon that can occur in a matter of hundreds of years instead of millions.

The area covering Polynesia consists of thousands of miles. It's interesting to note that two other groups of people live just outside of this area, and they have very different features.

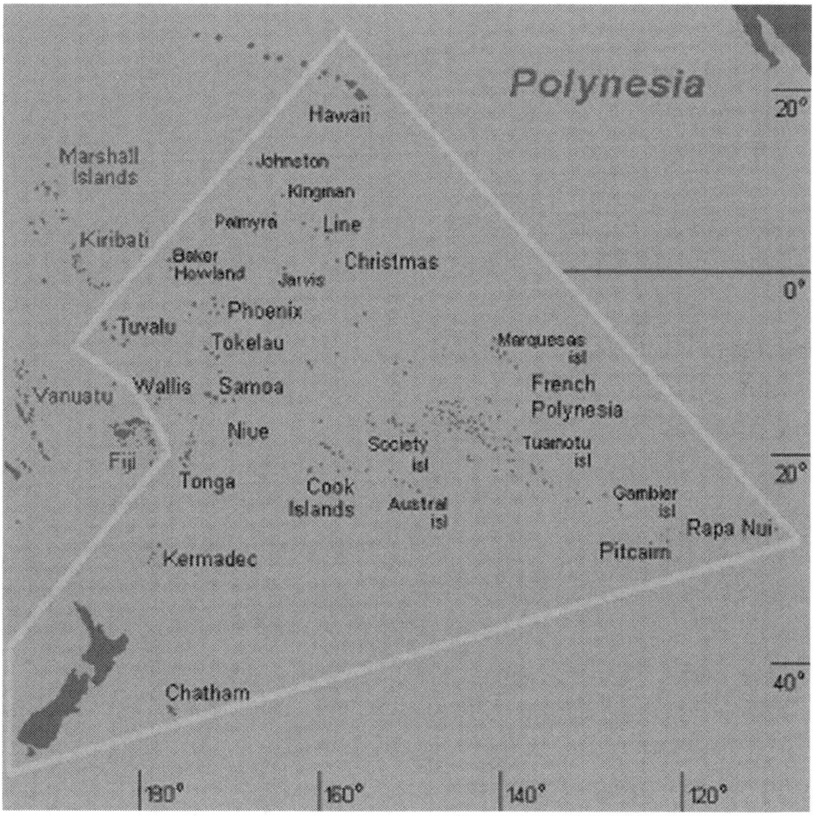

A wide area consisting of 24 major islands is home to the Polynesians. Fiji, which is not far from Samoa, is mainly occupied by the Melanesians. They have different characteristics from the Polynesians.

The three groups of people who live in the Pacific areas are the Polynesians, Micronesians and Melanesians.

Micronesians are the "pure" Austronesians. They physically look identical to Filipinos, with brown skin, straight or wavy hair and round eyes. They also have a very similar culture to Filipinos, especially since all of them were part of Spain for 300 years.

Melanesians are believed to be related to Papuans (of Papua New Guinea). They were one of the earliest branches of humanity to leave Africa, long before anyone else. They look African but are actually one of the most genetically distant branches of the human species from Africans.

The Melanesians probably originated from an Austronesian group that, over time, absorbed more Melanesian genes from Papuans through intermarriage. They have black, brown or blond hair that is very curly, and eyes that can range in color from dark brown to blue. They have very dark skin, hence the name Melanesian. They have more powerful builds than Micronesians, but are not particularly tall.

Polynesians are believed to be the more distant branch of Austronesians derived from mixing with the Micronesians and Melanesians. These are the "large" islanders. They inherited the larger muscle masses of Melanesians, but due to some odd chance of genetic mixing, they also ended up with high instances of physically larger builds. They inherited the curlier hair and larger noses of Melanesians, but retained the skin tone of Micronesians and most of their other features. A large physique was often considered attractive in Pacific Island societies—a mark of higher social status.

Polynesian people are mostly archipelagic people and they live as fishermen. Their dishes are mostly based on fish and coconut, which is abundant in the island ecosystem. Both fish and coconut have high protein and fat content. After many generations of eating such a high amount of fat and protein, their bodies adapted to become tall (determined by protein sufficiency) and big (determined by fat consumption).

In reviewing photos of old Hawaii and Samoa, I noticed that 100 years ago, most people were not as big today. It's probably because the people had to labor for their food, and their food was mostly unprocessed. The Pacific Island diet in the modern age tends to include a lot of meat (especially fatty mutton from New Zealand) as well as a lot of starchy foods and a substantial intake of salt. I was told that fresh fish in Samoa is much more expensive than the imported mutton or corned beef, and many Samoans simply cannot afford it.

It's a combination of factors including diet, lifestyle and culture—but the main culprit is globalization. Most of the Pacific Islands were traditional societies, dependent on subsistence farming and fishing until the mid-20th century. The arrival of U.S., French and British militaries during the Pacific campaigns of World War II began a colossal shift, as the islands opened up to the world.

The changes of the Samoan lifestyle didn't begin in earnest until the 1970s. The result was that the South Pacific had only about 40 years to adapt to a more modern, sedentary lifestyle. The islanders have now developed a taste for imported rice, sugar, flour, soda, beer and canned meats such as Spam, ham and corned beef, as well as frozen meats.

By studying the genomes of more than 5,000 Samoans, researchers have uncovered a single gene that boosts a person's obesity risk by upwards of 40 percent. Remarkably, this gene has most likely arisen in the population as the South Pacific was colonized.

As described in *Nature Genetics*, this "thrifty" genetic variant, called *CREBRF*, is associated with a 1.5% increase in Body Mass Index (BMI). So, for a person of average height weighing around 180 pounds, this gene is estimated to add an extra 10 pounds. As noted by the researchers in their study, *CREBRF* promotes more efficient storage of fat.

They also noted that the Samoan population has some of the highest obesity rates in the world, a fact that prompted the genetic investigation in the first place. Around a quarter of all Samoans involved in the study had the genetic variant, which was associated with 30–40% increased odds of being obese compared to those who didn't have the gene. At the same time, this gene is virtually non-existent in European and African populations and occurs at very low frequencies among East Asians.

"Although we have found a genetic variant with a reasonable biological mechanism, this genetic variant is just one part of the many reasons for obesity among Samoans," noted researcher Dr. McGarvey.

Other factors include diet and physical activity. Indeed, the globe's shift to calorie-rich processed foods and more sedentary lifestyles has contributed significantly to the elevated rates of obesity among Samoans. But as this new study points out, their genetics are also working against them.

The gene appears to work by causing cells to store more fat and release less energy. It's as if the cells are trying to conserve as much fuel as possible. The incidence of elevated levels of the gene among Samoans supports the evolutionary theory that only those who could conserve energy among early settlers survived the long journeys.

Now, Samoans no longer require this gene. Instead of being beneficial, it has become detrimental. Upwards of 80% of men and women in Samoa are now overweight.

Samoans weren't obese 200 years ago. The gene hasn't changed that rapidly, so the rise of obesity in Samoa cannot be blamed on this gene alone. The preference for processed food, a high carbohydrate and fat diet and a sedentary lifestyle have played even a bigger role than the gene.

Chapter 18
Samoan Warfare

WARS AMONGST THE SAMOANS were for a long time frequent and bloody. In fact, it was seldom the case that the islands were free from actual warfare or local quarrels.

Writing about the Samoans as he found them in 1830, Reverend John Williams, the first Western missionary to Samoa, explained, "The wars of the Samoans were frequent and destructive.... The island of Apolima was the first line of defense, a natural fortress of the people of Manono, a small but important island."

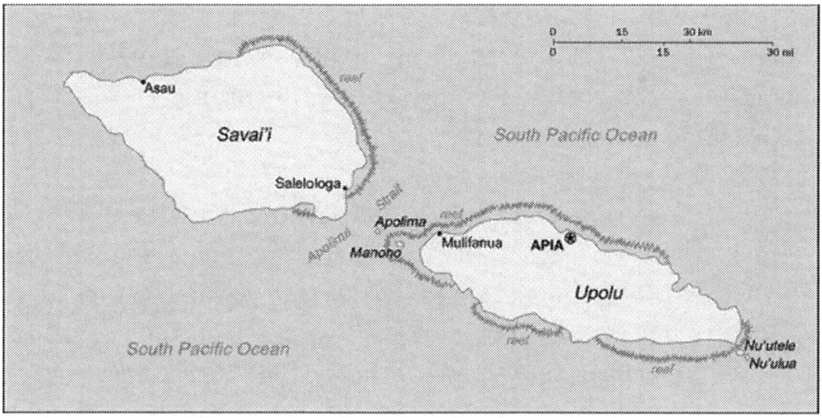

Two small islands between the two major islands.

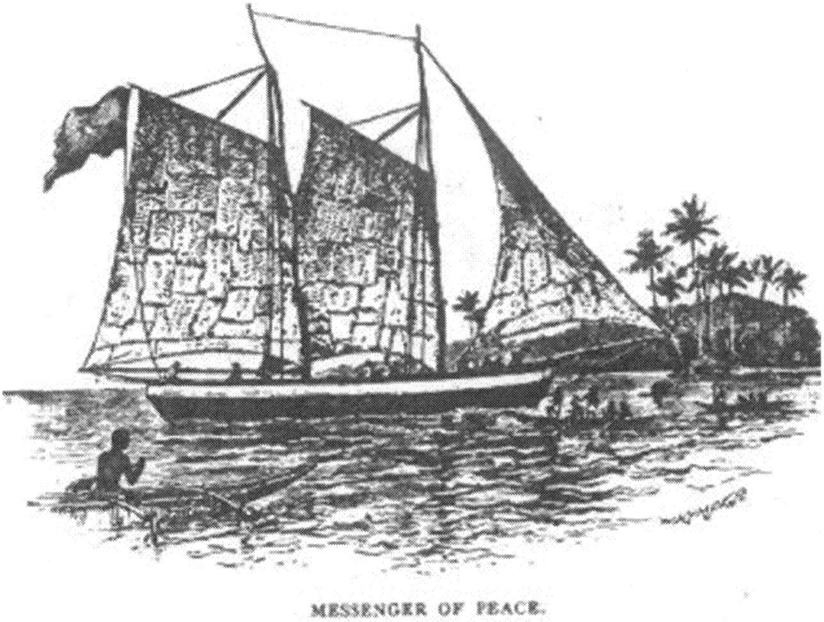

Messenger of Peace.

Reverend Williams arrived at Savaii in the Messenger of Peace in August, 1830, and anchored there in full view of dreadful fires and burnings on the shores of the island, on the opposite side of the straits, some thirty miles across. Recording the terrible scenes he witnessed, he wrote:

> *While we were engaged in lading the canoes to land the teachers, our attention was arrested by observing the mountains on the opposite side of the straits enveloped in flames and smoke; and when we inquired the cause of it, we were informed that a great battle had been fought that morning, and that the flames which we saw were consuming the houses, the plantations, and the bodies of women and children and infirm people who had fallen into the hands of the conquerors. Thus, whilst we were landing the messengers*

of the gospel of peace on the one shore, the flames of a devastating war were blazing on the opposite shore.

Below is John Williams's detailed account of the wars between the Samoan tribes:*

These people, although ignorant of the art of writing, kept an account of the number of battles they had fought, by depositing a stone of a peculiar form in a basket, which was very carefully fastened to the ridge of a sacred house appropriated to that purpose. This basket was let down, and the stones were counted whilst I was there, and the number was one hundred and twenty-seven, showing that they had fought that number of battles. And this was the list for one portion of the islands only! In this record, too, a stone was not placed after every conflict or battle, but simply at the close of each struggle or campaign, the stones being larger or smaller according to the duration of the conflict

Formerly the only arms used by the Samoans were clubs, axes, spears, and slings, but of late years firearms have been introduced, and generally adopted throughout the islands, whilst iron axes and knives have quite superseded the old stone axes and adzes. Clubs, spears, and slings are still used in warfare.

The sling was always considered a very formidable weapon, and old warriors have repeatedly assured me that a wound from a stone hurled from a sling and thrown with force was often much worse than one received from a musket-ball. If a stone struck the arm or leg, it was difficult to heal, since the bone was usually smashed to pieces, and caused much suffering.

---

* Excerpts reprinted under the *Creative Commons Share-Alike License*, from John B. Stair, *Old Samoa.* (Papakura: R. MacMillan, 1983). Part of the *New Zealand Electronic Text Collection.*

Wars originated from various causes, sometimes the most trivial. Amongst others were bad language, irritating songs, jealousy, quarrels relating to women, murders, political rivalry, and, in addition to these, old feuds, which frequently needed but the merest trifle to fan them into a flame. The pride of many chiefs was also a fruitful source of war and bloodshed, which evils were not simply occasioned by their intrigues to gain power, but also in some instances from a desire to have their name associated in the recollection of posterity with a war; it being the custom to enshrine the names of those more particularly connected with a war in the record of it.

When war was declared, messengers were dispatched in various directions to summon allies, who were requested to assemble at a given rallying-point on a certain day. If the war was between two districts, it commenced immediately, and even when more extensive operations were contemplated a small force often made a raid upon some portion of the enemy's territory without waiting for all the forces to assemble. Much effort was also made by both parties to strengthen themselves by fresh alliances, and in attempts to draw away forces from their opponents' allies. The assembled warriors were accustomed to hold a review and sham fight, at which time the various chiefs assembled to divide the battle, i.e. to appoint the post of duty to the different bands of warriors, and otherwise make arrangements for the battle.

Both sea and land forces were employed in combat, either separately or in combination. At times a division of a fleet of canoes was employed to make a sudden descent upon some portion of the enemy's territory, and having ravaged it, speedily to decamp, such attacks being usually made about dawn. Sea-fights were often bloody and destructive encounters.

As the fleets were approaching each other, the attention of the various crews was principally directed to the management of their canoes, whilst the warriors on the front part of each canoe strove to spear the helmsman of the canoe they were opposing. When the fleets neared each other the canoes often became locked, and then followed a desperate hand-to-hand encounter.

If the canoes were not entangled, most of the crews were at times more or less able to engage in the combat, leaving some of their number free to take charge of the canoes, and fill up the place of the helmsman in case he fell.

Before a regular attack commenced a conference took place between the hostile parties, when formal speeches were delivered on either side. Sometimes, the warring parties would agree to have single combats between chosen champions selected from either side.

Reverend Williams went on to describe some of the atrocities committed against the members of opposing tribes during warfare:

The onslaught was usually desperate, and the battlefield obstinately contested on both sides, much carnage being the result.

In all conflicts revenge seemed to be the ruling passion; hence blood was shed without remorse, captives not being so much thought of as slaughter.

Before an engagement, the women and children, with old and infirm people, were always conveyed to a place of safety, called an olo; and on either side, being vanquished, the conquering party made a rush to overpower the guard left in charge of the camp, and thus wreak their vengeance on the helpless creatures who might fall into their hands.

Thus, in case the enemy succeeded in surprising the camp before the inmates had time to escape, the captives were slaughtered without mercy by the conquerors, unless they were women they chose to carry off to their families, or individuals saved by their friends. Sometimes information was conveyed to the olo in time to allow the inmates to scatter themselves through the forest; but this often proved of little value, as they were soon pursued and captured, and if they did escape for a time it was but to endure protracted misery from famine and constant anxiety.

The refugees, as well as the vanquished warriors, often remained for weeks together roaming the forests and subsisting upon berries and wild fruit; since, although edible roots were plentiful in many places, the wanderers were unable to cook them, as lighting a fire at once betrayed their hiding-place. Unless they could find shelter in some friendly village, or were taken under the protection of relatives, the fugitives after a time surrendered themselves to the conquerors, preferring to risk their anger and falling by the club or spear of their enemies, rather than perish by the lingering death of starvation or the tortures of suspense.

Sometimes the olo was a cave in which the defeated army sought shelter from their pursuers. If the victors were able to discover the hiding-place of the refugees, they immediately collected firewood and piled it up before the cavern, to smother the hapless captives.

The evils of war were many, revenge, jealousy, hatred, and mistrust were fostered, families broken up, and continual insults offered to the conquered party. Their plantations were destroyed, their settlements burnt, and even if permitted to return to their lands they were never safe from insult, their houses being entered with-out notice and plundered at the will of their oppressors. Their wives and daughters were insulted and degraded, and on the occasion of travelling parties visiting the conquered settlement, the inhabitants were made to submit to humiliating insults, persons of rank being compelled to perform the most degrading and menial duties, which they dared not resist.

Mere boys from the dominant party were accustomed to affect the airs of their elders, and order old grey headed men to cook food for them, and in case of refusal an armed party quickly followed, to devastate the settlement and plunder its inhabitants. Sometimes the vanquished were directed to climb cocoanut-trees, gather nuts, and then descend the tree head foremost, holding the nuts—two at a time tied together—between the teeth.

On other occasions, they were compelled to dive for poisonous fish, and having found them, to throw them into the air and catch them in their hands, which were pierced with their sharp poisonous spines, and great agony occasioned. They were also compelled to bite poisonous roots that produced intense pain, causing the mouth to swell greatly. It was useless to refuse to submit to these indignities, a severe beating being certain to follow a refusal, or even any expressed reluctance to submit to this tyranny.

The slain on the battle-field were treated with much indignity. The heads of the vanquished were cut off and carried in triumph, and these, as well as the bodies of the slain, were taken to the settlements in proof of their prowess by either party, unless one party were crushed. These heads and headless bodies were afterwards given over to the children for further insult, who were accustomed to drag them about the settlements in triumph, and then to spear, stone, or mutilate them still further, as they might choose.

The captives from Fasito'otai were selected for the first offerings, and after them followed others in quick succession, night and day, early and late, until the last wretched victim had been consumed. Most heartrending were the descriptions I received from persons who had actually looked on the fearful scenes enacted there.

Innocent children skipped joyfully along the pathway by the side of their conductors and murderers, deceived with the cruel lie that they were to be spared, and were then on their way to bathe; when suddenly the blazing pile, with the horrid sight of their companions and friends being thrown alive into its midst, told them the dreadful truth; whilst their terror was increased by the yells of savage triumph of the murderers, or fearful cries of the tortured victims which reached their ears.

The Rev. S. Ella assures me that he was told in after years that four hundred victims were burnt there in that fearful sacrifice to revenge.

I found Reverend Williams's account of the Samoan wars most riveting, as well as sobering as to what humans could do to one another.

Chapter 19
The Samoan Language

ONE DAY A YOUNG NURSE at the eye clinic remarked to me, "Dr. Hung, I read that the Polynesians were originally from Taiwan. So I think we are related because the people in Taiwan are Chinese."

I smiled and replied, "Yes, it is truly a small world."

The nurse was only partially correct. Indeed, through DNA studies, scientists have proved that the Polynesians are related to the original indigenous people of the island of Taiwan. But they were not Han Chinese. The Han Chinese from the mainland only began arriving in Taiwan several hundred years ago, mostly from the province of Fujian across the strait from the island. Then in 1949, after the Kuomintang lost to Mao's communist takeover, millions of Han Chinese fled to the island. The original people of Taiwan were pushed further up into the mountains.

The original Taiwanese were believed to have come out of Southeast Asia, and they were related to the Malay race, the people now inhabiting Malaysia, Indonesia and the Philippines. The Malay and Polynesian languages belong to the same family—Austronesian.

Samoan, a Polynesian language, is the first language for most of the Samoan Islands' population of about 246,000 people. With many Samoans living in other countries, the total number of speakers worldwide was estimated at 510,000 in 2015. It's the third most widely spoken language in New Zealand, where 2.2% of the population, or 101,900 people, were able to speak it as of

2018. According to the Australian census of 2006, there were 38,525 speakers of Samoan in Australia at the time, and US Census 2010 showed more than 180,000 Samoans residing in the United States (triple the number of people living in American Samoa), presumably many of whom spoke Samoan.

Samoan was only a spoken language until the early to mid-1800s, when Christian missionaries began arriving in the islands. The first problem the missionaries faced was that of learning the language. The second was that of identifying the sounds in the local languages using the letters of their own languages to establish alphabets for recording the spelling of native words. Through this, the Latin script for writing was introduced, and in 1834, an orthography (conventional spelling system) of the Samoan language was distributed by the London Missionary Society. Having established more-or-less satisfactory alphabets and spelling, teaching the indigenous people how to write and read their own language was next. A printing press, with English alphabet keys, was part of the mission equipment, so it was possible not only to translate and write out portions of the Bible scriptures and hymns in the local language, but also to print them for use as texts in teaching. Thus, the missionaries introduced writing for the first time in Samoa.

The first complete Bible (*Tusi Pa'ia*, Sacred Book) in Samoan was completed and published in 1862. The same year, Reverend George Pratt, a missionary with the London Missionary Society who lived for 40 years in Matautu on the island of Savai'i, wrote *A Grammar and Dictionary of the Samoan Language, with English and Samoan Vocabulary*. The book contains sections on Samoan proverbs and poetry in addition to the grammar and dictionary entries.

The Samoan alphabet consists of only 15 letters: 5 vowels—a, e, i, o, u; and 10 consonants—f, g, l, m, n, p, s, t, v. In addition, a macron (*fa'amamafa*) written over vowel letters indicates the five long vowels, ā, ē, ī, ō, ū, differentiating words that otherwise share the same spelling, as, for example, in *manu* (animal) and *mānu* (float, afloat).

Loanwords from English and other languages have been adapted to Samoan phonology, which use the additional letters h, k and r:

/k/ is retained in some instances (Christ = *Keriso*, club = *kalapu*, coffee = *kofe*), and has become [t] in rare instances (such as *se totini*, from the English "stocking").

/d/ becomes [t] (David = *Tavita*, diamond = *taimane*, dollar = *tala*).

/g/ becomes [k] in some cases (gas = *kesi*).

/h/ is retained at the beginning of some proper names (Herod = *Herota*), but in some cases becomes /s/ (hammer = *samala*), and is omitted in others (herring = *elegi*, half-caste = *afakasi*).

/z/ becomes [s] (Zachariah = *Sakaria*)

/w/ becomes [v] (William = *Viliamu*)

/b/ becomes [p] (Britain = *Peretania*, butter = *pata*)

Some nouns are derived from verbs by the addition of either *ga*, *saga*, *taga*, *maga*, or *'aga*: such as *tuli* = to chase; *tuliga* = chasing.

Sometimes place is indicated by the end of a word: such as *tofā* = to sleep; *tofāga* = a sleeping-place, a bed.

The simple form of the verb is sometimes used as a noun: *tatalo* = to pray; *'o le tatalo* = a prayer; *poto* = to be wise; *'o le poto* = wisdom.

A few diminutives are made by reduplication: *pa'apa'a* =, small crabs; *pulepule* = small shells; *liilii* = ripples; *'ili'ili* = small stones.

Adjectives

Adjectives are made into abstract nouns by adding an article or pronoun: *lelei* = good, *'o le lelei* = goodness; *silisili* = excellent or best, *'o lona lea silisili* = that is his excellence or that is his best.

Some adjectives are primitive, such as *umi* = long; *poto* = wise. Some are formed from nouns by the addition of *a*, meaning "covered with" or "infested with"; thus, *'ele'ele* = dirt; *'ele'elea* = dirty; *palapala* = mud; *palapalā* = muddy.

Others are formed by doubling the noun, as in *pona* = a knot, *ponapona* = knotty; *fatu* = a stone; *fatufatu* = stony.

Adjectives that express colors are mostly reduplicated words: *sinasina* or *pa'epa'e* = white; *uliuli* = black; *samasama* = yellow; *'ena'ena* = brown; *mumu* = red, etc.

Syntax

The normal word order in Samoan sentences is verb–subject–object (VSO). The other three most commonly used word orders are:

subject–verb–object (SVO); verb–object–subject (VOS);
and object–verb–subject (OVS).

These are all examples of ways a Samoan might structure *The girl went into the house*:

VSO
Sa alu le teine 'i le fale.
Went girl house

SVO
Le teine sa alu 'i le fale.
The girl went house

VOS
Sa alu 'i le fale le teine.
Went house girl

OVS
Le fale sa alu le teine
House went girl

Similarly to the Chinese language, the order of words in a sentence can change its meaning.

Oratorical register (level of usage of a language)
The Samoan language is notable for the differences between formal and informal speech, as well as a ceremonial form used in Samoan oratory.

Historically and culturally, oratory—also sometimes referred to as "chiefly" or "dignified" speech—is an important form of the Samoan language. It incorporates classical Samoan terms and prose as well as a different set of vocabulary, which is tied to the roles of orator chiefs (*tulāfale*) and speechmaking (*failāuga*) that remains part of the culture's continuing indigenous *matai* system of governance and social organization. It's uncommon for entire conversations to be held in the chiefly level of speech. It is used mainly in making formal introductions between individuals, opening and concluding formal meetings and executing ceremonial tasks (such as the Samoa 'ava ceremony).

The *gagana fa'aaloalo* (polite speech) is used by lower-ranking people to address people of higher status, such as their family *matai* chief, government officials or clergy. It's also the formal level of speech used among chiefs during ceremonial occasions and social rites such as funerals, weddings, chiefly title bestowals and village council meetings.

It's considered proper to use the "polite" language when praying as well. Untitled people (those without *matai* chief titles) who are unfamiliar with each other will often greet each other in a chiefly or polite level of speech as a common courtesy, while familiar individuals frequently use chiefly addresses in jest (as in humorously addressing friends with *talofa lava lau afioga*—"respectful greetings your highness"—instead of the more colloquial *malo sole!*—"hey man!").

Below are some examples of "polite" word variants according to social rank:

English	Common term	In relation to a "High Chief"	In relation to a "Talking Chief"	In relation to a "Tufuga" artisan/builder
house	fale	māota	laoa	apisā
wife	to'alua, avā	faletua, masiofo	tausi	meana'i
dog	maile	ta'ifau	'uli	

Another form of speech in "polite" Samoan includes terms and phrases of self-abasement that are used by the speaker in order to show respect and flatter the listener. For example, when praising another woman's child, a mother might politely refer to her own children as *ui* (literally, "piglets"). To emphasize the beauty of a fine tapa cloth, the presenter might refer to it as a simple *vala* (plain cloth). The weaver of an especially fine mat might call it *launiu* (coconut leaf), in order not to appear boastful.

Overshadowing the dignity or prestige of higher-ranking individuals is a serious offense in Samoan culture. Words are chosen very carefully to express individual feelings in a way that acknowledges relative statuses within social hierarchy.

This form of self-abasement is also used in the Chinese language, such as referring to a person's own child as "my foolish son," and so on.

Numbers

The cardinal numerals are:

Numeral	Samoan	English
0	noa, selo (English loanword)	zero
1	tasi	one
2	lua	two
3	tolu	three
4	fa	four
5	lima	five
6	ono	six
7	fitu	seven
8	valu	eight
9	iva	nine
10	sefulu	ten
11	sefulu ma le tasi, sefulu tasi	eleven
12	sefulu ma le lua, sefulu lua	twelve
20	luafulu, lua sefulu	twenty
30	tolugafulu, tolu sefulu	thirty
40	fagafulu, fa sefulu	forty
50	limagafulu, lima sefulu	fifty

60	onogafulu, ono sefulu	sixty
70	fitugafulu, fitu sefulu	seventy
80	valugafulu, valu sefulu	eighty
90	ivagafulu, iva sefulu	ninety
100	selau, lau	one hundred
200	lua lau, lua selau	two hundred
300	tolugalau, tolu selau	three hundred
1000	afe	one thousand
2000	lua afe	two thousand
10,000	mano, sefulu afe	ten thousand
100,000	Selau afe	one hundred thousand
1,000,000	miliona (English loan word)	one million

The term *mano* was an utmost limit until the adoption of loan words like *miliona* (million) and *piliona* (billion). Otherwise, quantities beyond *mano* were referred to as *manomano* or *ilu*; that is, innumerable.

Similarities to Other Austronesian Languages

Despite the geographical distance, Samoan is closely related to other Malayo-Polynesian (i.e., Austronesian) languages, with many of them sharing some of the same words or root words, numbers and names of mythological gods.

Below are a few examples of words from 3 other Austronesian languages (Tongan, Hawaiian and Malay) that share similarities with the Samoan language:

English	Samoan	Tongan	Hawaiian	Malay
hello	talofa	malo e	aloha	
sky	lagi	langi	lani	langit
two	lua	uata'ifau	elua	dua
five	lima	nima	elima	lima

As you can see, the Samoan language wouldn't be too difficult to learn. In contrast to languages like Khmer or Thai that require a person to learn a new alphabet, the Samoan uses the Latin alphabet and phonetic spelling. In addition, the grammar is simple and the vocabulary limited, with many loan words that are usually borrowed from the English language.

Chapter 20

The Third Gender

ONE OF THE FIRST Hawaiian words I learned after arriving in the islands was *Mahu*, which I learned was synonymous with the drag queens who frequented the Hotel Street area in Honolulu. Because of the complaints from sailors and other visitors, the city government actually enacted a law that required these drag queens to wear a badge indicating that they were men. *Mahu* was also a derogatory term for a male homosexual. Later I learned that it was more than just the term for the above two.

Mahu ("in the middle" in Hawaiian) is broadly defined as men with feminine mannerisms or women who are trapped in men's bodies. There is evidence of their presence and social functions in ancient times in Polynesia.

The first published description of *māhū* occurs in Captain William Bligh's logbook of the Bounty, which stopped in Tahiti in 1789, in which he was introduced to a member of a "class of people very common in Otaheitie called Mahoo... who although I was certain was a man, had great marks of effeminacy about him."

Mahu in Native Hawaiian and Tahitian cultures are third gender people with traditional spiritual and social roles within the culture, similar to Samoan *fa'afafine,* Tongan *fakaleiti*, the Cook Islands Māori *akava'ine,* the Māori *whakawāhine,* the Niuean *fiafifine* (also *fakafifine*), the Tokelauan *fakafāfine,* the Tuvaluan *pinapinaaine,* the Gilbertese *binabinaaine,* and the Wallisian *fakafafine.*

This third gender is found in almost all Polynesian cultures.

On my first trip to Samoa, we were invited to party in a village not far from where John grew up. A boy of about thirteen with shoulder-length hair, who had feminine mannerisms and wore a red Hibiscus flower in his ear was dancing to the beat of the music. As I had read about the third gender people in the Polynesian culture, I asked a John if this boy was a *Mahu*.

"He is a *fa'afafine* or third gender," he replied matter-of-factly.

In Samoa, fa'afafine has been a part of island life for as long as anyone can remember. Most villages have *fa'afafine*, with an estimated several thousand across Samoa's islands.

The word *fa'afafine* includes the prefix fa'a–, meaning "in the manner of" or "way of," and the word *fafine*, meaning "woman." Strong evidence exists that points to Samoa existing under matriarchal rule for centuries before contact with Europeans. Queen Salamasina, holder of four paramount chief titles, ascended the throne by the shrewd maneuvering of the powerful female chieftains around her. Samoa had and continues to value the leadership roles of women and third genders. As such, there are no prohibitions in the past or present that bar the transfer of chiefly titles to women or *fa'afafine* and there is a long list of *fa'afafine* chiefs in the ancient past leading all the way to the present.

Fa'afafine are known for their hard work and dedication to the family, in the Samoan tradition of *tautua* or service to family. Ideas of the family in Samoa and Polynesia include all the members of a *sa*, or communal family, within the *fa'amatai* family systems.

In Samoa, there is very seldom ridicule or displeasure toward a biologically male child who states that they are a girl. For instance, one study showed only a minority of parents (20%) tried to stop their *fa'afafine* children from engaging in feminine behavior. Being pushed into the male gender role is upsetting to many *fa'afafine*. A significant number stated that they "hated" masculine play, such as rough games and sports.

A prominent Western theory among the many anthropological studies of Samoans was that if a family had more boys than girls or not enough girls to help with women's duties about the house, male children would be chosen as a substitute to be raised as *fa'afafine*.

Many of the *fa'afafine* in Apia interviewed regarding this theory thought it was nonsense and felt that no boy or man could be turned into a *fa'afafine* if they weren't born as such. According to some researchers, the existence of *fa'afafine* could be accounted for by a gene that directs altruism in an extended family. The theory proposes that androphilia (attraction to men or masculinity) could be passed down because it is advantageous to have non-traditional roles for some members in their society.

One of the chief proponents of the theory, Paul L Vasey, contends that the existence of androphilia may serve the evolutional purpose of providing support for related kin. This means that *fa'afafine* and other non-traditional roles, such as unmarried aunts and uncles, would have more time and resources to dedicate to the success of their kin. Freed from the constraints of a traditional marriage and the raising of their own children allows *fa'afafine* to excel in nurturing the family and community dynamics. This fits nicely in Samoan society where hierarchy is highly stratified and customs are strictly adhered to.

***

While working in Apia, I read about one of the more famous *fa'afafines* in Samoa in the local newspaper.

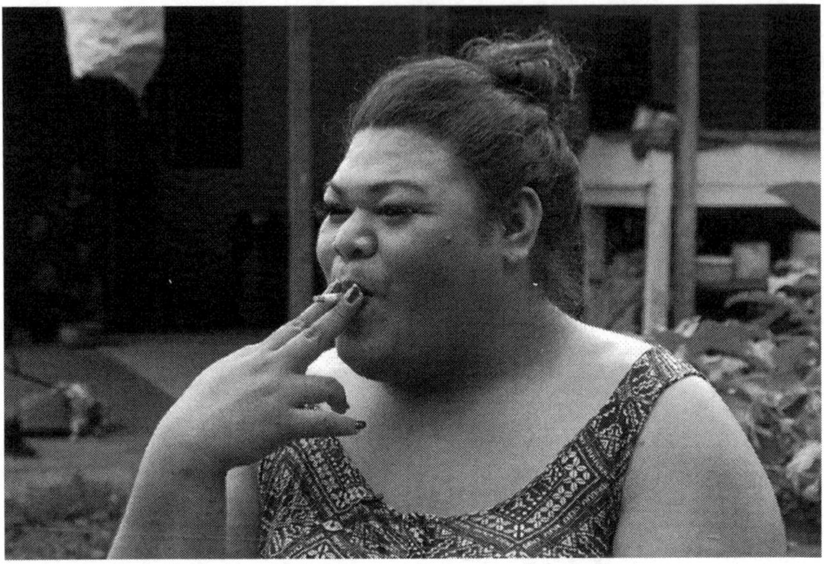

Keyonce Lee Hang, a well-known Samoan *fa'afafine*.
(Photo credit: Jonathan Barrett, Reuters)

The article* describes Keyonce Lee Hang—self-named after singer Beyoncé—preparing for a traditional lunch following church on Sunday and caring for her elderly grandmother. In addition to her duties at home and in the community, she works for the government's fisheries department.

She explains to the interviewer that the *fa'afafine* are widely misunderstood outside Polynesia and the South Pacific. "Western society tries to fit us [in] a box, to put us under gay, under trans and queer ... but I think fa'afafine is our cultural identity—it defines us."

* Barrett, Jonathan. *Samoa's 'third gender'delicately balances sex and religion.* July 30, 2019. Reuters.

Her mother says Keyonce began showing effeminate characteristics around the age of three, and would wear her sister's dresses. "Keyonce is my child and I accept my children as they are," she says.

The article goes on to explain that although most modern *fa'afafine* choose men as their partners, their cultural identity has nothing to do with sexual orientation. In Samoan law, sex between men is criminal and it's not socially acceptable for men to dress as women, but *fa'afafine* operate outside these parameters.

Although the church doesn't endorse same-sex relationships and considers them to be men, *fa'afafine* often lead church choirs and youth groups, and plan and decorate church events. Reverend Taufao, general secretary of the Congregation Christian Church in Samoa, tells the interviewer that *fa'afafine* used to wear more neutral clothing and often partnered with women, but he states that they are welcomed by the church.

Fa'afafine are valued in Samoan society as hard workers, particularly in leadership roles for charitable causes and as caregivers for people such as the elderly. A store owner in Apia points out to the interviewer that it can be an advantage to have someone who fulfills culturally female roles but who has a man's muscle.

***

The Samoa Fa'afafine Association (SFA) of independent Samoa, based in Apia, has been active for over a decade. It works closely with government, local churches, and youth organizations, supporting community projects for the *fa'afafine* community, and also for elders and youth in Samoa. The SFA has been active on the international level working with the United Nations and

Pacific regional NGOs, on behalf of the *fa'afafine*, transgender, and LGBT communities of the Pacific Islands.

This is another aspect of the Samoan culture I find interesting. It is truly an accepting society.

Chapter 21

The Aggie Grey's Hotel

IN 2017, I RECEIVED AN URGENT LETTER from my friend Peter Bonadelli in Samoa saying that Dr. Taloa had just unexpectedly quit her job as the only ophthalmologist in the entire country. Peter had been treated for eye problems himself, and he begged me to come to Apia to help out at the eye clinic, and also to treat his own eye conditions. As he was a prominent resident of Samoa, the head of a large NGO and on the board of a few others, I assumed he had consulted hospital authorities and they had asked him to contact me about working at the hospital.

Getting to Samoa from Honolulu, 2,200 miles to the north, hadn't gotten any easier since my last visit. The only Fiji Airlines flight still departed at 1 am, and was notorious for delays. I could have taken a Hawaiian Airlines flight to Pago Pago 100 miles away, but getting between Pago Pago and Apia was complicated and was also often plagued with delays. I was just grateful not to be sandwiched between two large Samoans, as I had been on another trip.

After being disappointed in 2014 that the Aggie Grey's was being rebuilt following cyclone and flood damage, I was thrilled on this trip to have accommodation at the hotel, which had reopened under the management of the Sheraton Hotel group. Being a gold member of the Sheraton Hotels, I was upgraded to an ocean view suite facing Beach Road.

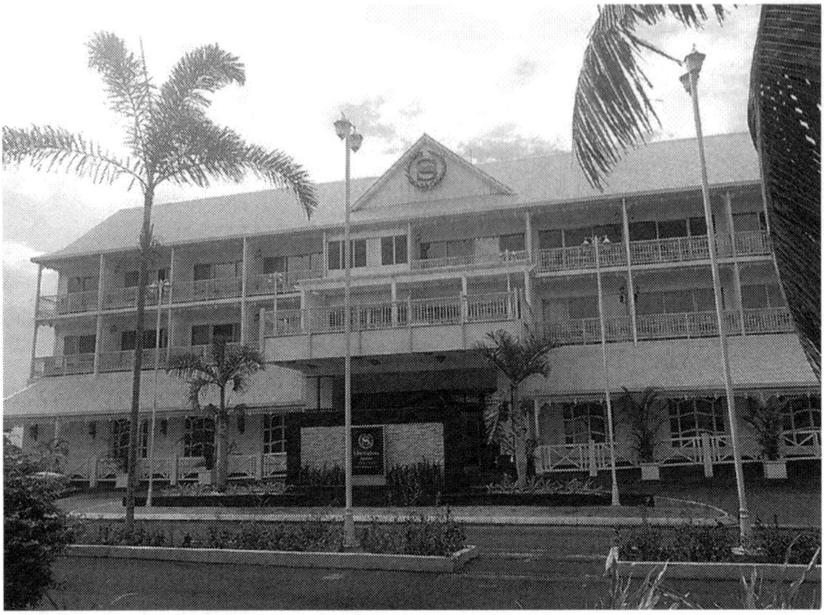

The Aggie Grey's Hotel in Apia, Samoa.

The Aggie Grey's Hotel & Bungalows is a historic hotel. It was opened in 1933 by Samoan entrepreneur Aggie Grey, and became a popular gathering place for American servicemen stationed in Samoa during World War II.

Many notable actors, including Dorothy Lamour, Marlon Brando, Gary Cooper, William Holden and Raymond Burr stayed at the hotel. It was involved with the production and housing of the crew on the American film *Return to Paradise* (1953) starring Gary Cooper.

The hotel in Apia is not to be confused with Aggie Grey's Lagoon Beach Resort, also operated by the Sheraton, on the north-west coast of Upolu, 30 kilometers (19 mi) west of Apia.

Aggie Grey was born Agnes Genevieve Swann in 1897, the daughter of British settler William Swann—the only chemist in Samoa for many years and a good friend of Robert Louis Stevenson's—and his Samoan wife Pele. In 1903 her mother died and Aggie was raised by her father and later by him and her step-mother.

Aggie Grey grew to be a pioneering figure of the Samoan hotel industry, and was one of the country's most popular and well-known figures. She was very active in the Samoan social scene, and became the subject of two biographies by Nelson Eustis and Fay Alailima.

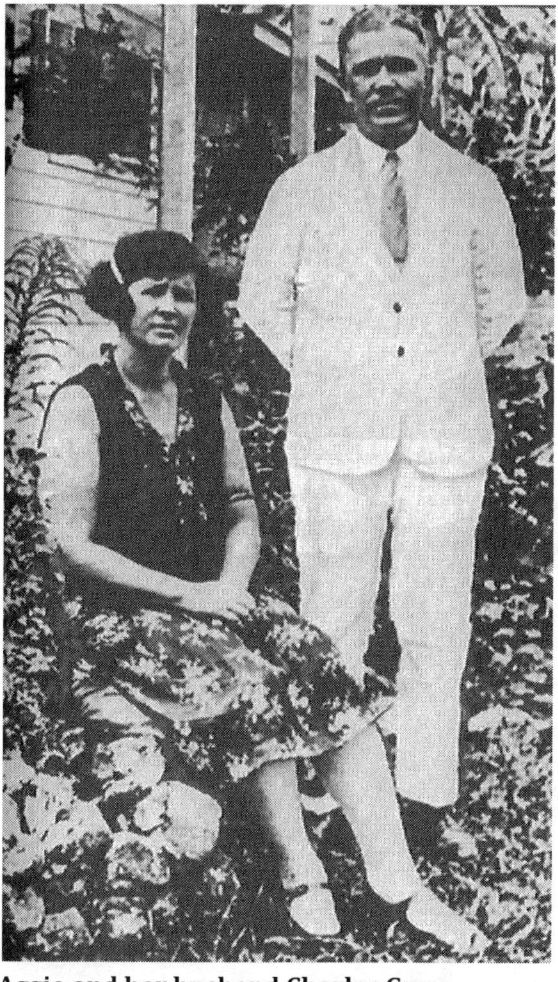

Aggie and her husband Charles Grey.

Aggie was friends with American writer James Michener and she and her sister Mary Croudace (Aunty Mary) were widely believed to be possible models for his character Bloody Mary in *Tales of the South Pacific* (1946). The book was adapted into the Broadway musical blockbuster *South Pacific* by Rodgers and Hammerstein in 1949 and subsequently into the 1958 film of the same name.

She died in 1988.

The Aggie Grey's Hotel has been a legend among generations of South Pacific travelers for its fabulous informality and friendliness.

In 1971, the Western Samoan government issued a stamp, one of a series promoting tourism, bearing a picture of Mrs. Grey and her picturesque, old-fashioned hotel's central building, a landmark at the eastern end of the curving Apia waterfront. The stamp gave the establishment, already famous in the South Seas, worldwide free advertising.

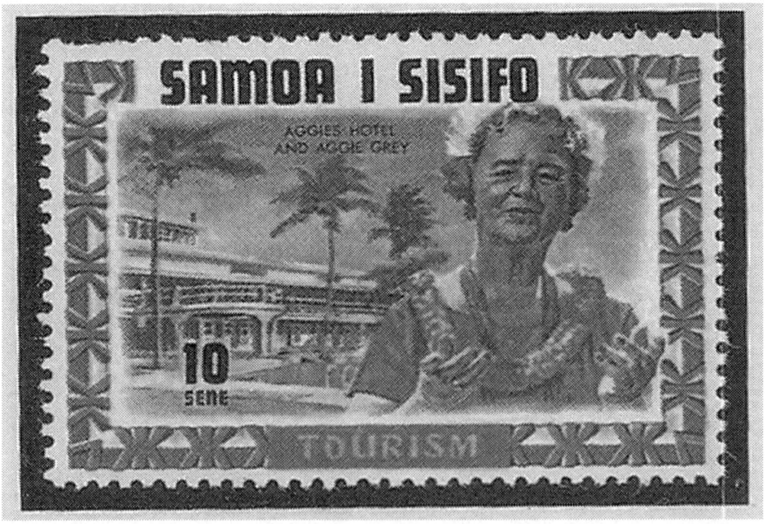

In 1971 Samoa honored Aggie Grey with a special postage stamp.

An Australian man in his nineties who had frequented the hotel over many decades told me that instant camaraderie was part of the charm that had drawn generations of South Pacific travelers back to Aggie Grey's Hotel. "It's hard to be lonely there," he explained.

He also told me that Aggie Grey herself had often surveyed the scene from a stool at the tiny serving counter. She had developed the quintessential South Seas inn of a bygone era, preserving the aura of the past, but with such modern amenities as air conditioning.

She developed the hotel from a sandwich stand catering to American servicemen stationed in Western Samoa during World War II. The decor is pure South Pacific Art Deco. The wood carvings and arrangements of seashells on the exterior walls and pillars are a mishmash of Polynesian and Melanesian themes unidentifiable with any particular island.

My room, in the main front wing, was spacious and had all the amenities of a five-star hotel. More elaborate accommodations were contained in the nearby cluster of separate cottages with thatched roofs, modeled after the traditional Samoan village house, or *fale*.

Most rooms were in the two-story wings that formed a quadrangle enclosing the large swimming pool and one giant *fale* that was used for the hotel's regular feasts and entertainment. The wings were new additions to the fabled main building, a white-painted wooden structure that resembled an old-time plantation-owner's mansion.

From the dining room in the old building, which also contained the lobby, there were views of Apia Harbor on one side and a tangle of tropical vegetation in other directions. The plantation atmosphere was enhanced by the daily pouring of afternoon tea, served free with cookies, on the broad veranda overlooking the luxuriant garden and pool.

The old timer also told me that tipping was discouraged, being considered contrary to the Samoan tradition of hospitality. But times had changed, and now waiters expected tips.

The huge festival *fale* had no walls, and consisted of a high thatched roof supported on poles of polished native hardwood in the traditional Samoan manner. It was described in hotel folders as "the biggest Samoan-style building in the South Pacific," and "the biggest nail-less building in the Southern Hemisphere."

Inside was a bar and long buffet tables for the almost nightly *fiafia*, or Samoan feast. The abundant food laid out for self-service included the favorite Samoan taro and coconut dish *palusami*. Other native dishes include suckling pig roasted in an underground *umu*, succulent local crab, baked fresh fish, baked taro, baked breadfruit and an assortment of exotic tropical fruits.

There were wooden chairs for visitors who found it uncomfortable to sit cross-legged on woven mats in the native fashion. The evening entertainment was furnished by a troupe of young singers and dancers recruited from the village just outside the hotel's grounds.

I had a wonderful, unexpected vacation, as after arriving in Apia, I found out that I wasn't needed at the hospital.

Unbeknownst to Peter Bonadelli, a young Samoan doctor named Akau, whose grandfather was Chinese, had just finished her eye training in Fiji and was hired to assume Dr. Taloa's position.

I offered my help, but she indicated that she was managing and would let me know if she needed me.

On the recommendation of one of the doctors, I went to the Samoan Circus Show one day. It was a circus without animals, mostly consisting of fantastic acrobatics. The show was very entertaining. The star attraction was the tallest man in the world, a Turkish man named Sultan Kosen who was 8 feet 3 inches tall.

A few weeks earlier in California, I had given a lecture on diabetes and endocrine problems, using acromegaly as an example of when a tumor in the pituitary gland secreted excess growth hormones and led to growth such Sultan's. I was interested to see him and take a picture with him so I could add the photo to my future lectures. He looked very uncomfortable standing up because he was so tall, and he had to sit down after just a few minutes.

The following day, I visited Manono Island. I hired a small boat to take me across to the island situated in the Apolima Strait between the main islands of Savai'i and Upolu.

It was one of the scariest boat rides I'd ever taken, as there were no life vests, and we were out in the open ocean. The small boat was continually splashed with water. I had never really learnt to swim for any distance. I thought I could probably save my own life only if the boat capsized within twenty feet from shore! The entire time I was on the boat, I worried that my wallet would get wet. I don't know why I had such a silly obsession, never mind that I could have lost my life if the boat capsized!

Once on solid ground, I walked around the island. I had a chance to experience the truly authentic Samoa, where many trappings of modern life, including traffic, were left far behind. It was truly a tropical paradise.

As I walked, I tried to imagine the first English missionary's accounts of the ferocious battles fought on this island.

Home to just four small villages, Manono is only 3 square kilometers (1.1 square miles) in size, and Samoa's third most populated island. Although it's just 4 km off the coast from Samoa's main island, Upolu, Manono Island seemed a world away. People lived and cooked according to thousands of years of tradition. Life was more traditional, and no cars or dogs were allowed there. It was so much more peaceful than the main islands.

I stopped by someone's house where a small café had been set up, and had a cup of coffee.

Before sunset, I got back on the boat and returned to the big island of Upolu.

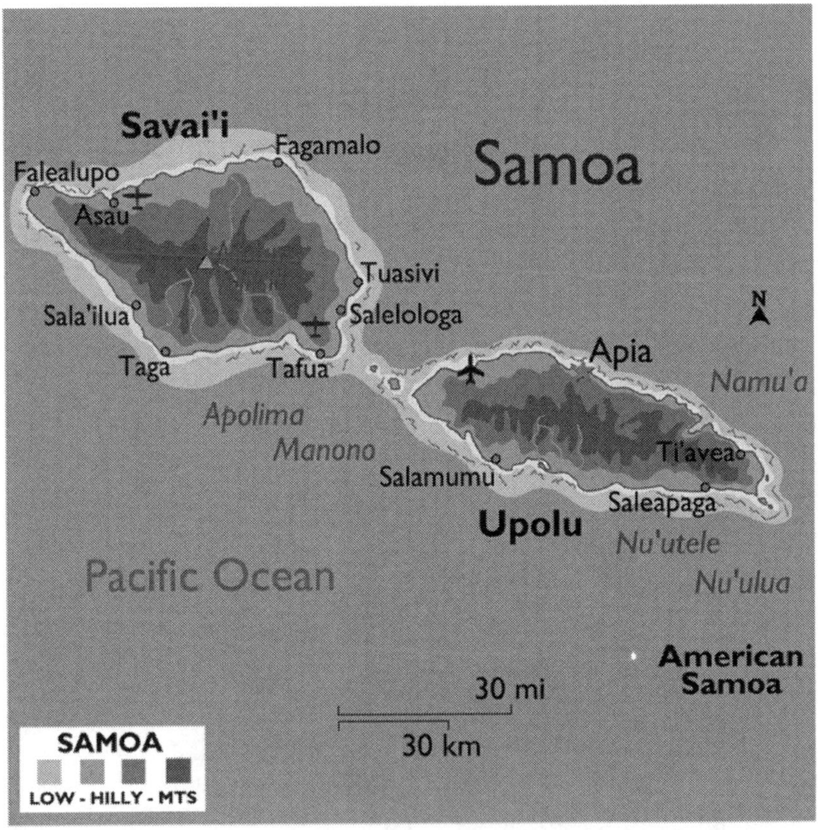

The two small islands of Manono and Apolima between the larger islands.

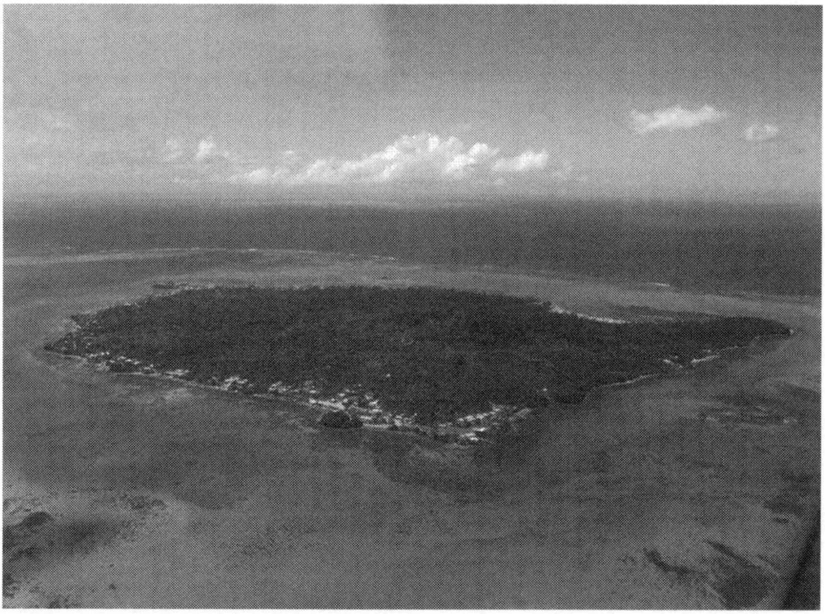

Manolo Island.

Sunday evening, I boarded Fiji Air and flew back to Honolulu.

My next project will be Vanuatu. My good friend Chua Huck Cheng's daughter Lynn and her husband David have been working in the country to advocate for the natives' health care, and she approached me to help with eye care there.

At the time of writing, Vanuatu was still closed to the outside world because of COVID. When it re-opens, I will head for that country.

I have already begun learning the Vanuatu language Bislama, which is an English-based creole language. I have found it amazingly simple and easy to learn.

I look forward to checking out Vanuatu and learning about the people and the country, and I hope to find the richness of experience that the Samoan Islands have given me. I will never forget the generosity and kindness of the Samoan people, and I am grateful for my dearly missed friend John, who started it all.

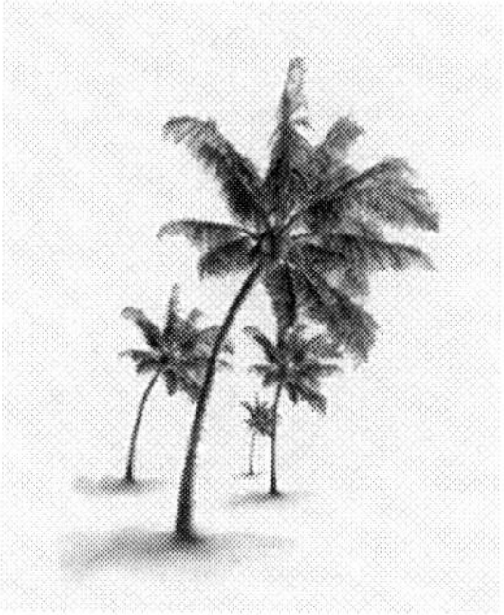

Made in the USA
Monee, IL
19 April 2026

48641209R00114